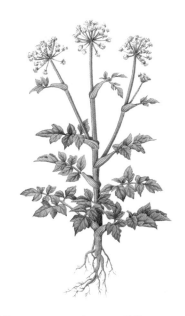

Health And Healing
The Natural Way

———————

Nature's
Medicine Chest

———————

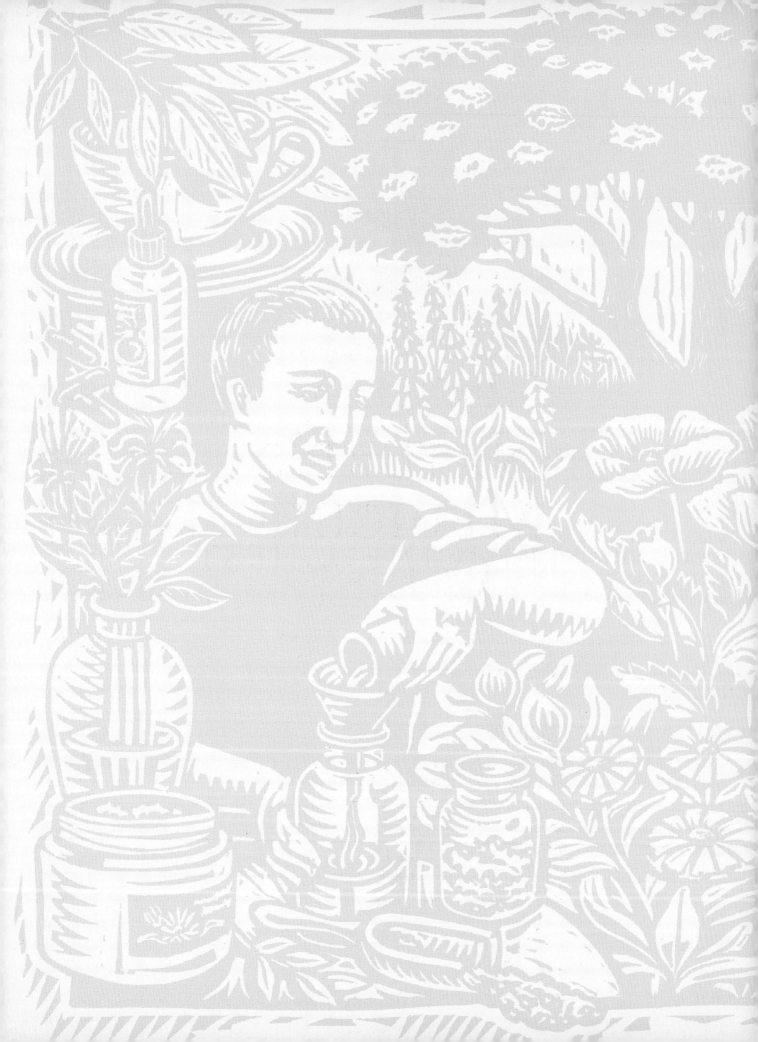

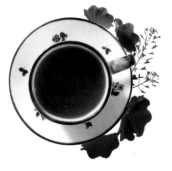

HEALTH AND HEALING
THE NATURAL WAY

NATURE'S MEDICINE CHEST

Reader's Digest

PUBLISHED BY

THE READER'S DIGEST ASSOCIATION LIMITED

LONDON NEW YORK SYDNEY MONTREAL CAPE TOWN

NATURE'S MEDICINE CHEST
was created and produced by
Carroll & Brown Limited
5 Lonsdale Road, London NW6 6RA
for The Reader's Digest Association Limited, London

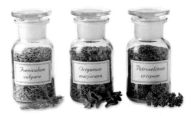

CARROLL & BROWN

Publishing Director Denis Kennedy
Art Director Chrissie Lloyd

Managing Editor Sandra Rigby
Managing Art Editor Tracy Timson

Editor Laura Price

Art Editor Gilda Pacitti
Designers Rachel Goldsmith, Jonathan Wainwright

Photographers David Murray, Jules Selmes

Production Wendy Rogers, Clair Reynolds

Computer Management John Clifford, Karen Kloot

First English Edition Copyright © 1997
The Reader's Digest Association Limited,
11 Westferry Circus, Canary Wharf,
London E14 4HE

Copyright © 1997
Reader's Digest Association Far East Limited
Philippines Copyright © 1997
Reader's Digest Association Far East Limited

ISBN 0 276 42266 X

Reproduced by Colourscan, Singapore
Printing and binding: Printer Industria Gráfica S.A., Barcelona

CONSULTANT

Christopher Hedley MNIMH
Medical Herbalist

CONTRIBUTORS

Julian Barker Dip. Phyt., MNIMH
Medical Herbalist

Mark Evans MNIMH
Medical Herbalist

Adrian McDermott BSc., MNIMH
Medical Herbalist

Sabine Rickert MNIMH
Medical Herbalist

FOR THE READER'S DIGEST

Series Editor Christine Noble
Editorial Assistant Chloë Garrow

READER'S DIGEST GENERAL BOOKS

Editorial Director Cortina Butler
Art Director Nick Clark

The information in this book is for reference only;
it is not intended as a substitute for a doctor's diagnosis and care.
The editors urge anyone with continuing medical problems
or symptoms to consult a doctor.

NATURE'S MEDICINE CHEST

More and more people today are choosing to take greater responsibility for their own health rather than relying on the doctor to step in with a cure when something goes wrong. We now recognise that we can influence our health by making an improvement in lifestyle – a better diet, more exercise and reduced stress. People are also becoming increasingly aware that there are other healing methods – some new, others very ancient – that can help to prevent illness or be used as a complement to orthodox medicine.

The series *Health and Healing the Natural Way* will help you to make your own health choices by giving you clear, comprehensive, straightforward and encouraging information and advice about methods of improving your health. The series explains the many different natural therapies now available – aromatherapy, herbalism, acupressure and many others – and the circumstances in which they may be of benefit when used in conjunction with conventional medicine.

NATURE'S MEDICINE CHEST introduces readers to the diverse and fascinating realm of medicinal herbalism. It gives a clear and concise guide to the ways in which herbal preparations can help to heal and relieve common health complaints. You will learn how to make and apply herbal remedies, and also discover which particular remedies are recommended for specific complaints, from the common cold to arthritis. There is a fascinating overview of ancient herbal wisdom, the worldwide growth and practice of modern herbalism, and how traditional remedies remain useful today. At the heart of the book is a fully illustrated A–Z guide to the most widely used healing herbs, with notes on dosage and preparations and any special cautions. *NATURE'S MEDICINE CHEST* can bring the benefits of herbs and herbal remedies into your life and home.

CONTENTS

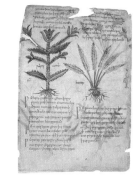

INTRODUCTION: HERBAL HEALING 8

1 THE CURATIVE POWER OF HERBS

DEFINING MEDICINAL PLANTS
AND HERBS 16

MEDICINAL PLANTS
THROUGH HISTORY 19

STUDIES OF AGE-OLD REMEDIES 25

HERBS AND PHARMACEUTICALS 27
The pharmacognosist 28

2 CURRENT USE OF HERBS

HERBS IN VARIOUS THERAPIES 32
The aromatherapist 34
The overstressed woman 37

HERBAL BEAUTY PRODUCTS 39
Making your own herbal face packs 41

THE FUTURE OF PLANTS AS MEDICINE 43
Using herbs for natural pain relief 45

3 USING HERBS SAFELY

FINDING AND PREPARING HERBS 48

CLASSIFYING HERBS BY USE 52

DANGEROUS HERBS 56

MISAPPLICATION AND
OVERDOSING 61

TREATMENT AND SELF-DIAGNOSIS 63
The indigestion sufferer 65

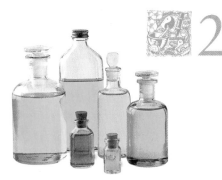

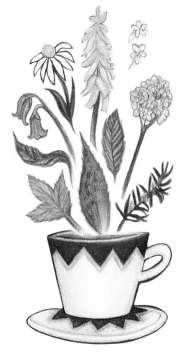

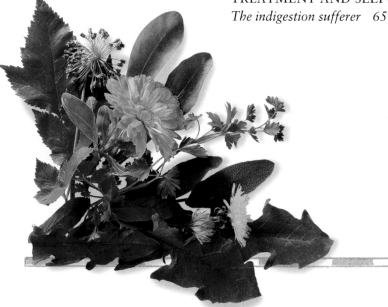

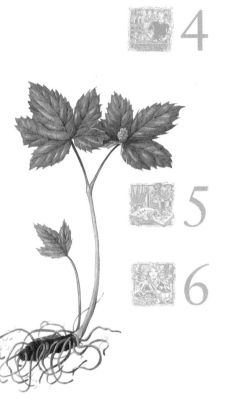

4 HERBAL PREPARATIONS

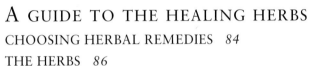

GROWING YOUR OWN HERBS 68
The horticulturist 70
Planting your own container herb garden 72
CUTTING AND DRYING HERBS 73
TYPES OF PREPARATION 75
Making your own inhalants 78
HERBS IN YOUR DIET 81

5 A GUIDE TO THE HEALING HERBS

CHOOSING HERBAL REMEDIES 84
THE HERBS 86

6 HEALING WITH HERBS

DIGESTIVE SYSTEM PROBLEMS 134
Using herbs to combat constipation 136
RESPIRATORY PROBLEMS 138
REPRODUCTIVE AND URINARY PROBLEMS 140
Painful period sufferer 141
HAIR AND SKIN PROBLEMS 143
The psoriasis sufferer 145
EAR AND EYE PROBLEMS 147
MOUTH, TEETH AND THROAT
PROBLEMS 148
HEADACHES AND MIGRAINES 150
MUSCLE PAIN 151
NERVOUS DISORDERS 153
The insomniac 154
AGEING PROBLEMS 155

INDEX 157
ACKNOWLEDGMENTS 160

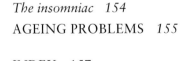
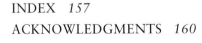

HERBAL HEALING

An insight into the age-old traditions of herbal remedies can help you to enjoy the powerful medicinal value of plants.

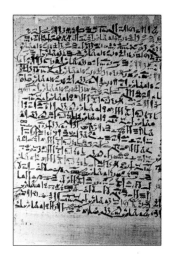

CULINARY MEDICINES
Many staple foods also have medicinal applications, although these are not necessarily achieved through ingestion. Cabbage leaves and potato juice can both be used as poultices to relieve swelling and tenderness. Other plants which bring relief include strawberries for sunburn, cucumber for itchy skin, lemon for chilblains and onion for bee stings.

EGYPTIAN HEALING
References to herbal remedies, some still used today, have been found in ancient Egyptian texts.

Herbs have been recorded in the earliest writings and have played a part in the evolution of human societies all over the world. The ancient Egyptians used herbs for embalming and the Bible refers to herbs, such as frankincense and myrrh, being used cosmetically and medicinally. North American shamans used herbs in their healing, as did the Chinese, Persians, Aborigines and other ancient peoples. However, conventional medicine, particularly in the West, is only just beginning to recognise the real medicinal value of the majority of common herbs.

Despite the growing importance of herbalism today, there appears to be no clear definition of a herb. Some definitions focus on the medicinal properties of the plant and others on culinary uses. Nevertheless it seems that most people agree that a herb is a plant used, whole or in part, as a medicine, a flavouring for foodstuffs, or as an aromatic or chemical addition to cosmetics. Such definitions, however, opens the term 'herbalism' to a great many geographical and social interpretations.

HERBALISM THROUGH HISTORY

For most of history and for the majority of the world's cultures there has been no strict delineation between plants that were used for healing and those that were used for food. All societies lived off the land and, by necessity, a variety of local plants made up part of their diet. It is hardly surprising, therefore, that people everywhere developed their local flora medicinally.

Around the world, healers have worked with a whole range of herbs and herbal preparations, endeavouring to treat any illness that presented itself. Inevitably, some of these early treatments proved to be ineffective and even dangerous, yet many survived to the present day and are still recommended as herbal remedies.

The earliest extant records of herbal medicine are believed to have been written by the Chinese emperor Pen T'sao who lived around 2500 BC. One thousand years later the *Ebers Papyrus* was written, containing over 700 references to herbs, many of which are still used today. Other peoples, most notably the Aztecs, American Indians and Persians understood the medicinal value of herbs as long ago as 1000 BC.

In Europe, the Greeks and Romans furthered the ancient knowledge of herbal remedies and much of their learning survived unaltered into the Middle Ages. The advent of the printing press brought with it the first medical and herbal books which were among the earliest books to be printed, and up to the 16th century, herbalism was by far the most widely-practised form of healing and medicine in Europe.

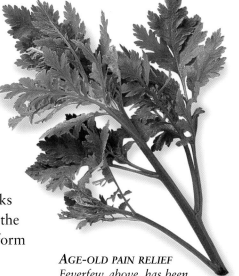

AGE-OLD PAIN RELIEF
Feverfew, above, has been used since the Middle Ages for its analgesic properties. Culpeper (see page 23), recommended the herb for 'all pains in the head' and current research has proven the efficacy of feverfew in relieving the pain of migraines and headaches.

WITCHCRAFT AND THE DECLINE OF HERBALISM

Healers have always held a position of power in society, whether those societies were ancient, modern, simple or complex. Many healers practised herbalism to a greater or lesser degree and were renowned and respected for their herbal knowledge.

Despite this, many 16th and 17th-century female healers and midwives were singled out for persecution during the famous witch-hunts of that time. This may have been due to their conspicuous role in society, but may also have been because of their use of herbal preparations. Many herbs widely used medicinally were also thought to be used for occult purposes. If the healer's potions and concoctions did not succeed as cures, they may have been viewed as poisons or deliberate acts of ill-will.

Even the harvesting of herbs was believed to change their powers for good or for evil. Some herbs used for their medicinal properties were picked during a full moon to improve their healing powers. Those used in witchcraft were supposedly more malignantly powerful when harvested as the moon waned. Some of the most poisonous herbs known were believed to have been used in the witches' flying potion and were therefore seen as doubly related to mysticism and the forces of evil.

Herbs also played a protective role in superstitious beliefs, however, and not every herbalist and healer suffered at the hands of the witch hunters. Rue (*Ruta graveolens*) was believed to hinder acts of witchcraft and diminish the potency of spells and hexes, while garlic (*Allium sativum*) is a well-documented protection

WITCHES' BREW
Witchcraft, magic and healing have long gone hand-in-hand. For centuries potions and preparations have been equated with the summoning of spirits, the capturing of souls and the power of flight.

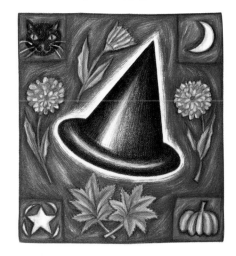

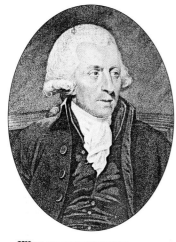

***WILLIAM WITHERING
(1741-1799)***
Withering heard tell of a selection of herbs that were used to cure dropsy. Rather than experimenting with the mixture as a whole, he tested each herb in turn and discarded all but foxglove.

ACTIVE PLANT MATERIALS
Research into the effects of plants on the body have led to the use of many natural remedies such as nasturtium leaves, below, which are a natural antibiotic.

against vampires. When the terror of the witch-hunts waned there grew a more scientific and less superstitious approach to the art of healing and the power of herbs.

MODERN HERBALISM

The break from traditional folklore towards a more scientific approach to herbs was aided by a growth in chemical and botanical understanding and advances in the tools used for analysis. This approach began early in the 19th century and many herbalists consider it to have started in earnest with the discovery and extraction of substances such as quinine from the cinchona tree. With these advances, scientists began to explore the effects that plant-based chemicals had on the human body while at the same time trying to identify the micro-organisms that invade the body causing diseases such as malaria. These two areas of research came together as herbal properties were employed in the battle against disease, and knowledge of the medicinal value of plants finally began to find its place in the medicine of the day.

In 1785 the English physician William Withering discovered the positive effects that foxglove (*Digitalis purpurea*) had on heart failure. He examined local herbalists' claims that foxglove leaves would cure dropsy – water retention – and recognised dropsy as a symptom of heart disease. His experiments showed that the foxglove did indeed relieve the effects of heart failure. Today, one of the most potent and widely-used heart stimulants – digoxin – is derived from the foxglove.

HERBS UNDER THE MICROSCOPE

The chemical analysis of plant matter over the past century has revealed many active constituents that we now know are responsible for the physiological effects of herbal, and many conventional, remedies. These active ingredients, including vitamins, minerals, saponins and tannins, have all been found to affect various parts of the body, thus helping to protect against, and give relief from, many disorders. Tannins, for example, have been found to effectively draw the cells of the skin together. This creates a stronger barrier against infection.

Using this knowledge of the effects of herbal ingredients allows herbalists to apply specific herbal remedies to disorders in relative confidence of the outcome.

As a form of healing, herbalism has gained growing respect among practitioners of conventional medicine and among those who have benefited from herbal treatment, and its popularity is now established throughout the world.

PROFESSIONAL HERBALISM

In the last fifty to sixty years the role of the professional herbalist has grown in the Western world. Although there are many drugs currently prescribed by doctors that have active constituents derived from herbs, there has been a gradual movement away from the often harsh and side effect-inducing drugs of conventional medicine. Improvements in the modern chemical industry mean that herbal extracts are more pure and more accessible than previously, and the popularity of over-the-counter herbal remedies in the West continues to grow.

A herbalist believes in a holistic approach to healing – treating the cause of the disease and the person as a whole rather than just the symptoms of the disease – and therefore needs to study a patient in some detail to prescribe precisely those herbs that will give the most benefit. Professional herbalists also give detailed advice to the individual with regard to curing and relieving general health problems and with information on herbs and their actions.

Although a professional herbalist will have access to more herbs and more specialised information than a person treating themselves with herbs, the growing respect for herbalism has increased the interest in and availability of self-help remedies.

HERBS AND HEALTH

Most herbal remedies are simple to make and straightforward to apply. Both internal and external applications can be taken in several forms, depending on the active ingredients you wish to use, and can invariably be made at home with basic kitchen equipment. Many herbs have water-soluble and alcohol-soluble constituents which have different effects on the body and are prescribed for particular ailments. Thus, a herb's water-soluble constituents may be utilised when taken as a tea or decoction, while a tincture will bring out the alcohol-soluble ones. It does not necessarily follow that any preparation of that herb will be equally useful so, when treating yourself, always monitor both your symptoms and your remedies.

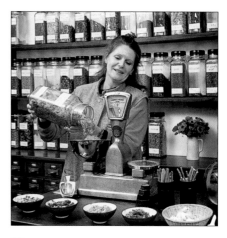

HERBALISM TODAY
Modern herbalists today have gained recognition in the East and the West, and medicinal herbs are now sold freely in high-street shops and marketplaces.

HOME HEALING
The increased interest in herbalism and the greater degree of available information has led to many people making and applying herbal remedies, such as the tincture below, at home.

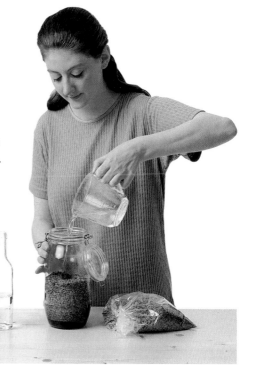

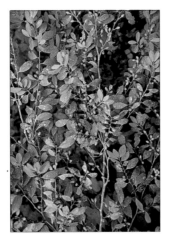

COCA PLANT
Many plants have been found to have specific chemical derivatives. One of the most widely known is the illegal stimulant, cocaine, derived from the coca plant, above.

KITCHEN CURES
Most herbal preparations are easy to make and simple to use. The honeysuckle syrup, shown below, offers fast and effective relief from sore throats and is simple to make at home.

HOW TO USE THIS BOOK

The purpose of *Nature's Medicine Chest* is to unravel and expose the facts and fiction of herbal healing. Chapter 1 offers a working definition of medicinal plants through history and looks at herbs as drugs and herbs as foods. This encompasses studies of age old remedies from around the world, and how the pharmaceutical industry has evolved from the study of plants. The chapter then explores the pharmaceutical preparations made from herbs today and the differences in preparation, action and use between herbal remedies and other drugs.

In Chapter 2 the current use of herbs in various therapies from herbalism and homeopathy, and in the make-up of household products, is discussed. The growth of herbalism highlights the importance of the rain forests of South America and their vast wealth of untapped healing. A brief look at genetic engineering and the role it plays in finding new natural medicines and 'designing' plants with higher quantities of healing properties concludes the chapter with a glance at the future of herbal remedies.

Using herbs safely is a very important part of home herbalism and in Chapter 3 you will discover how to find and prepare your herbs, where to buy or pick them and how to assess their quality, how best to store herbs to keep them fresh and how to prepare remedies without destroying the herbs' therapeutic properties. Here too you will find the properties of different parts of a herb and discover which herbs are best for home use and which are unsafe, and the dangers of self-diagnosis and overdosing.

If you'd rather grow, harvest, dry and prepare your own herbs, Chapter 4 gives all the advice you need, from planning a garden to applying your homemade cream. In Chapter 5 you will find over 85 common medicinal herbs listed in alphabetical order under their Latin names. Each entry includes a botanical description for the herb with its history, active ingredients, recommendations for use and, where necessary, cautions and contraindications.

Illnesses that respond well to herbal self-treatment are discussed in Chapter 6 where you will find all the details you need for relieving many common and specific ailments. If you have a complaint and wish to use herbs to treat it you can turn straight to Chapter 6 for proven remedies.

WHAT ARE HERBAL REMEDIES?

Many plants contain substances that affect the body's systems. When these plant extracts are used to treat illness or disease, the treatment is deemed a herbal remedy. To use herbal remedies to their best effect, it is important to understand the nature of the remedies and to make and apply them safely.

Q **WHERE DID HERBAL MEDICINE COME FROM?**
No-one can truly answer this question because one of the oldest uses of herbs that has been discovered dates back to prehistoric times. It is possible to state, however, that herbalism is thousands of years old and has been used by the most advanced and creative civilisations ever known. For many people the term herbalism may conjure images of druids or witches concocting magic potions, undermining any belief in the medicinal efficacy of the remedies themselves. In the past century the claims made for herbs in healing have come under increased scientific scrutiny and an amazing number of remedies have been proved effective.

In Chapter 1 you will find a wide-ranging history of the medicinal use of herbs, details on their current uses, scientific progress that is being made in the advancement of herbalism, and a glance at the future of healing with herbs. Chapter 2 focuses on the use of herbal preparations in various healing therapies such as aromatherapy and massage and the many common products that contain herbal extracts.

Q **HOW DO HERBAL REMEDIES WORK?**
The plants that are most widely used in herbal remedies contain many active therapeutic constituents that act upon the body. Such actions, whether gentle skin toning or causing sudden vomiting, can be harnessed and applied to relieve illness and disease. Some herbs have been used medicinally for thousands of years, but the extent of their therapeutic use may only recently have come to light. Echinacea, for example, has long been used to fight infections such as colds and flu, but current research into its immune-system-boosting effects has raised hopes that it may prove useful in the treatment of HIV and AIDS. For information on the active constituents of herbs and the physiological effects these have in fighting disease, see Chapters 4 and 5.

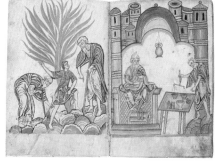

HERBAL HISTORY
Early herbals such as Dioscorides' famous book De Materia Medica *help us to understand the widespread history of herbalism.*

FUTURE HERBAL REMEDIES
The flowering tops of fresh hawthorn, shown below, are currently being researched for their therapeutic effects in relieving heart problems.

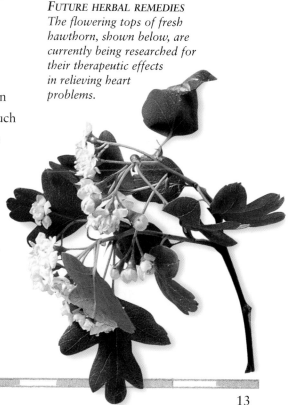

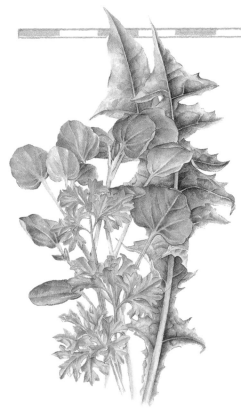

SUPER SALADS
There are some herbs that are recommended to be taken regularly even when you are not ill, such as those that are rich in iron and vitamins. These include salad herbs such as watercress, parsley, and dandelion.

TEA TONIC
A cup of warm skullcap tea taken three times a day can help to relieve and reduce the severity of headaches.

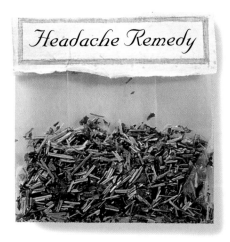

Headache Remedy

Q WHY WOULD YOU SEE A HERBALIST NOT A DOCTOR?
The simple answer is that you would not. Few therapists would ever suggest that you discard the help and advice of your doctor and turn solely to herbalism to cure all ills. This is not because they doubt the efficacy of the treatments, rather that the more complete treatment a person receives, the better. Most herbalists would recommend that a GP be kept informed of herbal treatments and some may even work with your doctor to provide the most effective treatment. There are, of course, certain disorders and situations where professional medical treatment should be sought, and your herbalist would never deter you from this. For details on such disorders, see Chapter 3.

Q IS HERBAL MEDICINE SAFE?
Natural herbal remedies are widely considered to be less harmful to the body than chemical drugs and tend to have a gentler yet equally effective action. With any treatment, however, it is vital that you understand the limits of the actions. There are several highly toxic herbs growing wild and even those not considered poisonous should still be taken with caution. Overdosing on herbal remedies is quite possible, and certain treatments are deemed unsafe for certain people. The diversity of actions a single herb can have means that, although you may take the remedy quite safely for indigestion, a pregnant woman or hypertension sufferer may experience dangerous side-effects. It is important, therefore, to be aware of the cautions and contraindications and to follow any guidelines carefully. Details for the safe application of herbal remedies can be found in Chapter 3 and in the individual entries in Chapter 5.

Q WHAT DISORDERS CAN HERBAL REMEDIES TREAT?
The majority of disorders a herbalist is asked to treat tend to be chronic rather than acute. This may be because many people feel more confident treating acute infections, such as tonsillitis, with antibiotics. In fact, herbal remedies are just as effective as many chemical drugs and, because they do not suppress the symptoms, will not mask an acute problem and turn it into a chronic one. Apart from the occasions listed in Chapter 3 when herbal remedies are not advised, there are numerous disorders that a herbalist can treat effectively. In Chapter 6 you will find a large number of ailments which will respond well to herbal remedies that you can make and apply at home.

CHAPTER 1

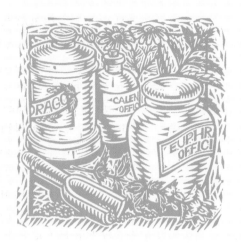

THE CURATIVE POWER OF HERBS

Herbs and other plants have been used to alleviate and cure illnesses since prehistoric times. Advances in medical and scientific knowledge have proved the efficacy of many of the traditional plant remedies, and some are at the forefront of conventional medicine today.

DEFINING MEDICINAL PLANTS AND HERBS

A herb may be both a food and a medicine depending on the way it is used, and many plants with medical properties are also common foodstuffs.

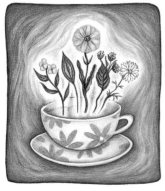

TEA THERAPY
One of the most popular medicinal uses of herbs is as a tea. Teas made from herbs such as peppermint and camomile can aid digestion as well as being refreshing.

It is not possible to draw an absolute line between medicinal and domestic plants and herbs. Peppermint, for instance, makes a refreshing cup of tea but is also used to relieve nausea. Professional gardeners and botanists use the term 'herb' to describe a herbaceous plant as distinct from a woody plant, that is a tree or a shrub. According to this definition, however, Linden blossom or oak leaves, which are used in herbal medicine, are from trees, not herbs. Yet carnations, for example, would be called herbs in horticulture even though they do not have medicinal uses.

HERBS AS DRUGS AND HERBS AS FOODS

If you pour boiling water on the fermented leaves of *Camellia sinensis* you usually do it because you enjoy the taste of the resulting drink and feel better for drinking it. You are, in fact, 'making a cup of tea'; a domestic and often social event which most people would say has nothing to do with medicine. We may not call the cup of tea 'medicine' but the boiling water extracts chemicals from the plant material which produce the welcome effect on the body.

Many people enjoy camomile tea – an infusion made by pouring boiling water on the flowerheads (or more likely a camomile tea bag) – either for its taste or relaxing effect. Few people, however, consider its medicinal properties – if you have eaten rather too well or too late in the evening, a camomile infusion can soon ease your discomfort and may also promote a restful night's sleep. Although camomile is both a domestic beverage and a medicine, taking it does not call for the advice of a professional

Fennel can be used as an antidepressant to lift mood

Marjoram acts as a circulatory stimulant and helps to relieve circulation problems

Parsley can be chewed to help to combat bad breath

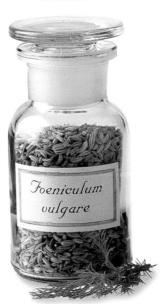

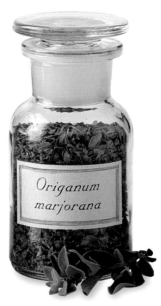

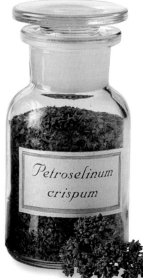

CULINARY CURES
Few people are aware of the therapeutic effects of many common kitchen herbs. With proper care and caution the same herb you use to flavour your cooking can be used in a more concentrated form to relieve pain or lift your mood.

Foeniculum vulgare

Origanum marjorana

Petroselinum crispum

any more than taking an aspirin would call for a doctor's advice, and self-medication, in this instance, is perfectly safe. Similarly there are herbs which are commonly eaten with food, either in fresh or dried form, such as parsley, basil, marjoram, oregano, mint and thyme which also have medicinal properties. They aid digestion and may contribute quite considerably to the nutritional quality of the meal. The minerals and vitamins which these herbs provide are essential to health but are needed little and often so there is no nutritional advantage in taking large amounts; indeed, if you ate the same amount of these herbs as of potatoes, for example, you would be at risk of being poisoned. In between the culinary amount and the toxic dose lies a useful medicinal dose: all of the herbs mentioned have uses besides flavouring your meals.

A food plant like lemon is treated much like a herb; it is a valuable source of vitamin C and while safe to consume in large quantities, most people find it too bitter – here taste, rather than toxicity, limits intake.

Many foods can also act medicinally when applied topically. Raw cabbage leaves, for example, help to relieve swollen arthritic joints and cabbage juice has been found to stimulate the digestive enzymes of the stomach; raw potatoes likewise make a useful poultice and, provided they have no green discoloration, the consumption of their juice can ease stomach pain. It is interesting to note that, apart from its tuber which we eat, the potato plant is poisonous with no therapeutic value. Indeed, its close relatives – deadly nightshade, henbane and thorn apple – are all very poisonous plants whose administration is restricted by law.

PHYTOMEDICINALS

While the medicinal value of some herbs can be experienced by eating the herb, others need their properties extracted using solvents. These resulting pharmaceutical preparations are called phytomedicinals – from the Greek for plant medicines.

Although some herbs like feverfew are only efficacious in their fresh state, the majority of medicinal herbs are used dried. The process of drying preserves the herbs and makes them easier to store, and removing the water concentrates the herb, making its effect stronger.

Once a herb has been dried, a solvent must be used to preserve it and extract the active ingredient. The most common solvent is alcohol. Many plant constituents will not dissolve in anything under 25 per cent alcohol and much higher percentages of alcohol are needed to dissolve resins (found, for example, in marigolds). The use of alcohol may vary depending on the intended application. If marigold is being used for its wound-healing properties an extract from the plant will be made using 90 per cent alcohol. To treat influenza, however, a herbalist would not use alcohol at all as the antiviral constituents are water soluble.

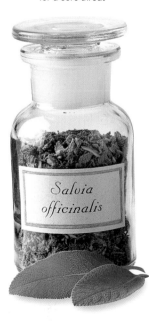

Sage has antiseptic properties and makes an effective gargle for a sore throat

Salvia officinalis

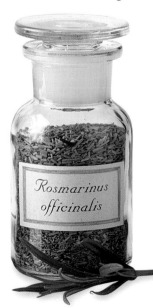

Rosemary is a warming circulatory stimulant that can lift mood and relieve fatigue

Rosmarinus officinalis

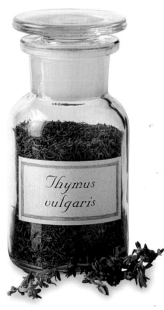

Thyme has an expectorant action and can be used to relieve chesty coughs

Thymus vulgaris

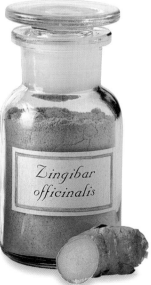

Ginger is a strong circulatory stimulant with anti-inflammatory and anticoagulant actions

Zingibar officinalis

SOME TRUTHS ABOUT HEALING HERBS

It is a fallacy that herbs cannot harm, only heal. Strychnine – one of the most highly poisonous plants and long used as an arrow poison – was once considered an effective painkiller. However, the tiny fatal dose and the fact that there is currently no known antidote made it too deadly for general medicinal use.

It is also not necessarily true that all natural herbs are superior to synthetic drugs. Although herbs tend to have a gentler action, they may also contain impurities. Treatment of stomach ulcers using liquorice may produce side effects such as hypertension because it contains glycrrhizin. However, a useful liquorice-based ulcer drug causes no side effects because the glycrrhizin is removed.

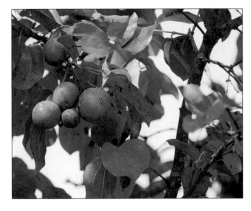

STRYCHNINE
Strychnine (Strychnos toxifera) *is one of the most poisonous plants in the world. It contains alkaloids which cause paralysis of the central nervous system and the lethal dose is extremely small. All parts of the plant are extremely poisonous.*

Other solvents

Glycerol and propylene glycol are sometimes used for medicines in cases where the presence of even a small quantity of alcohol is deemed undesirable, but they have their limitations as to solubility and may also hinder absorption within the body.

Other solvents used in the industrial production of medicines include methyl and propyl alcohols, acetone, ether and chloroform, which must be removed before the herbal extract can be sold or applied.

DIFFERENCES BETWEEN HERBS AND OTHER DRUGS

Although herbs are the basis of many drugs, there is a clear difference between the way a herbalist looks at a herb and a pharmacist looks at a drug. A herb in the sense that herbalists use it means whole-plant material, fresh, dried or extracted. The material may be from leaves, flowering tops, flowers, fruits, seeds, stems or underground organs such as roots, rhizomes, corms and bulbs, or it could be a product obtained by distilling whole-plant material such as volatile oils, or a product exuded by the living plant – such as juices, gums, latex and resinous material, usually from the bark of a tree. Even just one herb is a mixture of many active ingredients and herbalists frequently prescribe complex mixtures of herbs.

A drug in the sense that pharmacists – and, for that matter, the general public – use means a single compound with well-defined therapeutic goals.

Most drugs are presented in the form of a preparation to be swallowed, like a tablet or a capsule, or applied to the skin, like a cream, or introduced into a cavity of the body in the form of ear-drops or suppositories, for example.

Besides the drug itself, the preparation will contain fillers – such as chalk or lactose – which have no pharmacological use but may aid digestion or mask unpleasant tastes. Some drug preparations also contain a combination of two or three drugs, as in the case of many creams and the combined contraceptive pill.

DID YOU KNOW?

Some people believe that whole herbs are always more effective than their isolated constituents that are used in medicinal drugs. However, two of the most widely used and reliable heart stimulant drugs, digoxin and digitoxin, are more potent than the foxglove leaf from which they are extracted, a fact that is true of many herb-based pharmaceutical drugs.

HERBAL PAINKILLER
The opium poppy has been used for centuries as a painkiller and is still one of the most effective analgesics known.

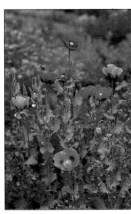

MEDICINAL PLANTS THROUGH HISTORY

In all places where humans have lived, plants have grown alongside them. Indeed, no known human society has ever existed without using plants for health and to treat illness.

One of the earliest known uses of plants, other than as food, was discovered at a Neanderthal burial site in a cave in Northern Iraq, where the remains of a man interred in flowers was unearthed in 1975. Carbon-dating estimates that the burial took place 60 000 years ago.

Ancient civilisations around the world, such as those in Papua New Guinea or the Amazon jungle, have an intimate knowledge, built up over thousands of years, of the plants that surround them and upon which they depend for their survival. Many of the herbal remedies they use today were probably also used by their Stone Age forefathers thousands of years ago.

It is also known that advanced civilisations based upon the agriculture of maize, peppers, squash and beans flourished at least 3500 years ago in Central America and Peru and their use of medicinal plants was extensive. These ancient uses of plants, and the fact that herbal remedies are still used worldwide today, gives some insight into the importance of plant life to man's existence from the earliest times.

THE LEGENDARY HEALERS

Most civilisations have healers of renown, whether real or mythological, a fact that spans centuries and continents, and links the power and fame of the healer with the growth of the society. Imhotep, the first recorded Egyptian healer, was physician to the Pharaoh Zoser just under 5000 years ago. It is difficult to separate his powers of astrology and magic from his use of plants, but his ability to heal has remained in the legends of that country for millennia. The Greek god of healing, Asclepius, may have actually lived before being assumed into a deity. The maxim: 'first the word, then the herb . . . and only then the knife' is ascribed to him. His daughter, Hygeia, was goddess of health in Greek mythology.

The ancient Greek physician Hippocrates – perhaps the most famous healer of all, and still known as the 'Father of Medicine' – paid great attention to the medicinal use of herbs, as well as to other factors such as diet and hygiene, in promoting health and preventing disease.

The Hippocratic corpus, which lay out Hippocrates' code of medicinal practice, was written in the 5th–4th century BC. Just like doctors, newly qualified herbalists in Britain today still swear an undertaking based upon the Hippocratic oath before acceptance into the National Institute.

The East

The earliest existing artefacts from Eastern herbalism are dated rather later than those in the West. The famed Chinese classical

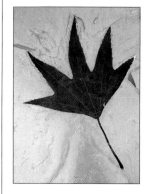

PREHISTORIC HERBS
Archaeological sites all over the world have provided fossils of plants, such as the leaf above from the Eocene era found in Utah, USA. These fossils help to trace the development of plant life to the present day.

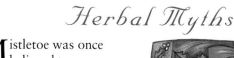
Herbal Myths

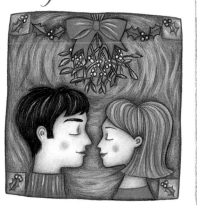

Mistletoe was once believed to grow where lightning had struck an oak tree. Druids saw mistletoe as the female essence to the oak's male principle which may have led to the sexual and fertility symbolism which still lingers today in the Christmas tradition of kissing beneath it.

pharmacopoeia, *Tzu-I Pên Tshao Ching*, is thought to have been composed in China about 500 BC, perhaps a little after the time of Confucius. The original contained 365 herbal remedies to which 200 were added later. Around the same time, *Susruta-Samhita*, the oldest medical text of India, was compiled, coinciding with the life of Buddha (560–480 BC). It names over 700 medicinal plants, arranged according to the condition to be treated. It is apparent, however, that the medicinal use of herbs was a well established practice in the East long before the creation of these texts.

In the Middle East, Crateuas (120–63 BC) was physician and herb collector to Mithridates, the ruler of Pontus. This herbalist-king was obsessed with the fear of being poisoned and focused much of his research on medicinal plants into the study of poisons and the search for antidotes.

The Biblical era

Many herbs and plants mentioned in the Bible are particularly noted for medicinal use and religious observation. In Psalm 51, for example, you can find the words 'Purge

me with hyssop and I shall be clean'. The Hebrew word 'ezob' in the original text is traditionally translated as hyssop, an aromatic plant which is believed to have medicinal properties, and it is almost certain that purification in the religious and medical senses were not distinct. Other scholars argue that the psalmist had a marjoram in mind – one closely related to the plant used today for upper respiratory infections.

Another example can be seen in Exodus 30:34: 'And the Lord said unto Moses, take unto thee sweet spices, stacte and onycha and galbanum: And thou shall make . . . a confection after the art of the apothecary,

A herbal time-line

This time-line illustrates the steady, worldwide interest that humans have had in herbs for the past 60 000 years. Trace the growth of herbal discovery from prehistoric man to the beginning of modern herbalism.

c. 60 000 BC
Neanderthals buried with herbal tributes. Pollen analysis of the flowers in a Neanderthal burial site in Northern Iraq identified nearly all of them as being still in use today. They included yarrow, mallow and grape hyacinth.

Alchemilla millefolium

2700 BC
Imhotep (above), the earliest recorded Egyptian physician, promoted carob, date, fig, olive, peach, pomegranate, garlic, lotus and lettuce as healthy foods with medicinal uses.

2500 BC
The earliest Sumerian herbal written. Almonds, apricot, poppy, turmeric, sesame and myrrh were all respected medicines. Their names were taken from the Sumerian into modern languages, indicating the great age of their use.

1500 BC
Advanced civilisations based upon the agriculture of maize, peppers, squash and beans and with an extensive use of medicinal plants flourished in Central America and Peru.

1500 BC
The Egyptian Ebers Papyrus presented a written compilation of prescriptions, most of them of plant origin, arranged according to the condition to be treated.

1000 BC
Asclepius, the Greek mythological hero who became a god of healing, may have lived as a celebrated herbalist and healer.

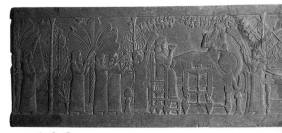

600 BC
Babylonian tablets (above) found in the ruins of the library of Nineveh describe a core of herbal remedies of about 200 plants.

560–480 BC
Susruta-Samhita, the oldest medical text of India, was compiled.

Melissa officinalis

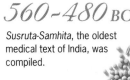

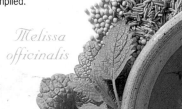

tempered together, pure and holy.' Stacte is still used as an incense in Catholic churches today. Onycha is a rockrose which exudes a gum later mentioned as medicinal by the Greek physician Dioscorides. Galbanum is an aromatic gum-resin that may have had medicinal uses and some members of the galbanum family are used in cooking today.

The later Classical Period

Three of the most famous herbalists of all time lived during the first centuries AD. Roman scholar Pliny's monumental *Natural History*, written around AD 77, dealt with medicinal plants. It abounds in errors but is lively and interesting. He pointed out rather shrewdly that the reason that herbal medicine was not better appreciated in educated circles was that it was known best by illiterate herb gatherers, and those who did have knowledge refused to pass it on for fear of losing their source of income.

Dioscorides was born in Greece in AD 40 and was probably a doctor in the Roman army. He travelled extensively and prided himself that his knowledge of plants was by direct observation in the field and from diligent enquiry from local sources. The plants in his *Materia Medica* are arranged according to medical usage.

Galen was born in Asia Minor in AD 130. He was a renowned physician in his day and became personal physician to the emperor Marcus Aurelius towards the end of his life. He put his considerable reputation behind the writings of Dioscorides, which is probably why they survived into the Middle Ages. Galen was highly critical of doctors who relied on apothecaries and herb collectors for their medicinal plants and took pride in his own practical abilities in the field. Ironically, the excellence of his work encouraged later generations to rely on the 'book-learning' he so deplored. The term 'galenical', still used today, refers to certain pharmaceutical preparations of plants.

The Middle Ages

After the fall of Rome, Classical learning was preserved by the Byzantine Greeks together with the great Arabic civilisation which emerged in the seventh century and swept across North Africa to Spain, bringing with it a golden age of Persian medicine.

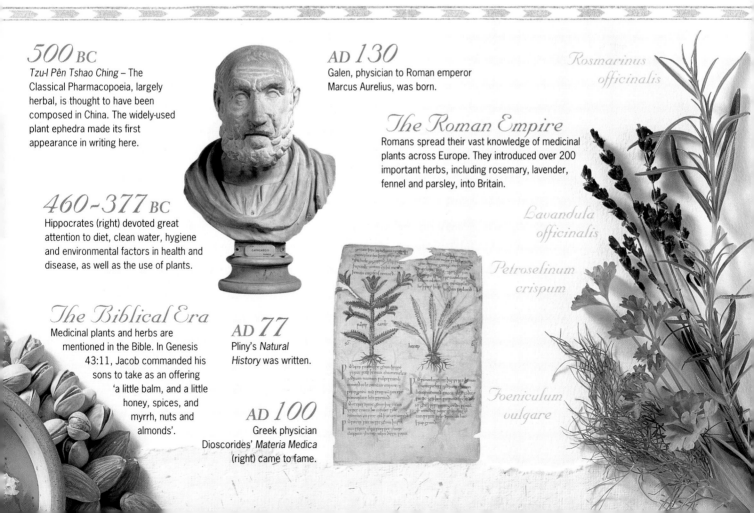

500 BC *Tzu-I Pên Tshao Ching* – The Classical Pharmacopoeia, largely herbal, is thought to have been composed in China. The widely-used plant ephedra made its first appearance in writing here.

460~377 BC Hippocrates (right) devoted great attention to diet, clean water, hygiene and environmental factors in health and disease, as well as the use of plants.

The Biblical Era Medicinal plants and herbs are mentioned in the Bible. In Genesis 43:11, Jacob commanded his sons to take as an offering 'a little balm, and a little honey, spices, and myrrh, nuts and almonds'.

AD 77 Pliny's *Natural History* was written.

AD 100 Greek physician Dioscorides' *Materia Medica* (right) came to fame.

AD 130 Galen, physician to Roman emperor Marcus Aurelius, was born.

The Roman Empire Romans spread their vast knowledge of medicinal plants across Europe. They introduced over 200 important herbs, including rosemary, lavender, fennel and parsley, into Britain.

Rosmarinus officinalis
Lavandula officinalis
Petroselinum crispum
Foeniculum vulgare

The great Persian physician Rhazes (Abú Bahr Mohammad ibn Zakarijá ar-Rázi) lived from about AD 865 until 925. He added greatly to the works translated from the Greek. As well as his many textbooks on medicine, he also wrote vast numbers of prescriptions; for colic he prescribed camomile, fennel, fenugreek and the seeds of quince, just as a herbalist might today.

Across Europe in the 10th century, a medical school was established at Salerno near Naples. Taking the best of Greek learning and Arab medicine, it flourished for 300 years and graduates earned the title 'Doctor'.

In northern Europe the Anglo-Saxons showed a keen interest in herbalism and a number of fascinating manuscripts have survived, combining herb lore with magic rather than science. They appear to have borrowed their basis for herbalism from the Physicians of Myddfai – a group of Welsh healers – who have been lauded for keeping alive classical medicine at this time.

One of the most famous medieval names in herbalism is St Hildegarde (1098–1179), Benedictine Abbess of Rupertsberg near Bingen, Germany. She wrote two medicinal books – *Physica* and *Causae et Curae* – and made the earliest known mention of some north European medicinal plants.

During the middle of the 13th century, Albertus Magnus, a remarkable German botanist and physician, wrote seven books on plants. As a Dominican monk, he was charged with inspecting each of their monasteries. This he did on foot, observing the plants along the way.

At the end of the Middle Ages the Swiss alchemist and healer Paracelsus wrote many tracts on herbalism. His first interest was in the alpine plants of his native land but later he recorded the plants used by gypsies and itinerant folk-herbalists. Although full of errors, his work signalled the gradual trend away from using whole plants to the 'single-ingredient' medication of the 19th and 20th centuries.

The Renaissance and beyond

The scientific vision of the ancient Greeks was revived in northern Italy during the Renaissance. By the 16th century this had helped to give rise to many herbalist-doctors all over Europe. During the early part of the

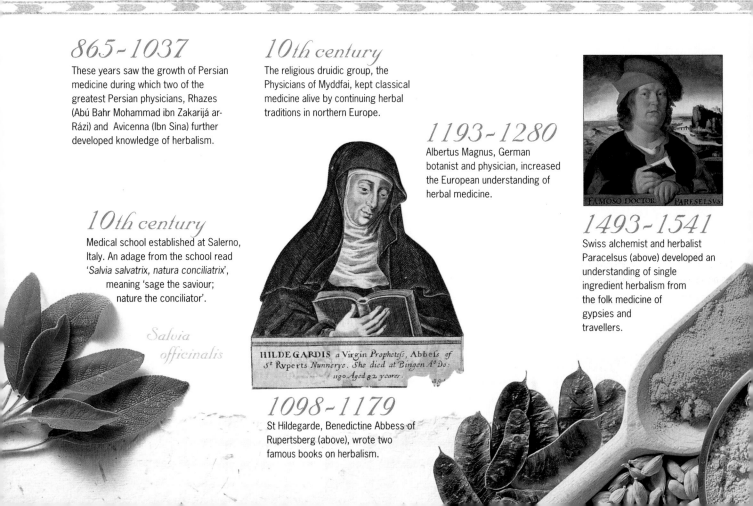

865–1037
These years saw the growth of Persian medicine during which two of the greatest Persian physicians, Rhazes (Abú Bahr Mohammad ibn Zakarijá ar-Rázi) and Avicenna (Ibn Sina) further developed knowledge of herbalism.

10th century
The religious druidic group, the Physicians of Myddfai, kept classical medicine alive by continuing herbal traditions in northern Europe.

1193–1280
Albertus Magnus, German botanist and physician, increased the European understanding of herbal medicine.

10th century
Medical school established at Salerno, Italy. An adage from the school read 'Salvia salvatrix, natura conciliatrix', meaning 'sage the saviour; nature the conciliator'.

Salvia officinalis

1493–1541
Swiss alchemist and herbalist Paracelsus (above) developed an understanding of single ingredient herbalism from the folk medicine of gypsies and travellers.

HILDE GARDIS a Virgin Prophetess, Abbess of St Ruperts Nunnerye. She died at Bingen A° Do: 1180. Aged 82 yeares.

1098–1179
St Hildegarde, Benedictine Abbess of Rupertsberg (above), wrote two famous books on herbalism.

16th century, Leonhart Fuchs (1501–85) wrote his masterpiece, *De historia stirpium*, which was noted not only for its keen eloquence but also for the superb woodcuts. He gave the name digitalis to foxglove, and fuchsias were named after him.

Around the same time, a doctor's son called Mathiolus (Pierandrea Mattioli) was singled out by the success of his written works. These started as commentaries on Dioscorides but progressed to superbly illustrated studies of all the plants known to him. It is said that the early editions of his *Commentaries* sold 32 000 copies.

Physicians from Flanders did much to stimulate and develop plant science. The plant genus *Lobelia* was subsequently named in honour of one of them – Lobelius (Mathias de l'Obel, 1538–1616).

The English herbalist John Gerard borrowed (to put it charitably) some of the text and most of the woodcuts from Continental sources for *The Great Herball or Generall Historie of Plantes*.

John Parkinson (1567–1650), 'herbarist' to Charles I, was the first to record some of the more useful medicinal plants native to Britain, such as the Welsh poppy and lady's slipper, a beautiful orchid which is now extremely rare.

Nicholas Culpeper (1616–54), one of England's most famous herbalists, was severely criticised in his own day for his complete reliance on astrology in his definition and examination of herbs. Two of his books – *Physicall Directory* and later *The English Physician* – were enormously popular, and have remained so to this day. An important part of Culpeper's appeal was doubtless his genuine compassion for the sick and his dislike of physicians who would rather import an expensive medicine from the East than use equally effective local plants.

CIVILISATIONS WITH ORAL CULTURES

Civilisations in North America, Africa and Siberia that did not develop a written form of language certainly knew herbal medicine and developed both theory and practice for their application which was passed down from generation to generation. Usually, as was the case in Babylon and ancient Egypt, the function of the doctor was combined

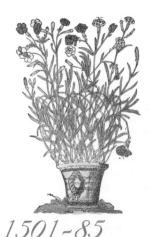

1501~85
Leonhart Fuchs wrote and illustrated (above) his masterpiece *De historia stirpium*.

1538–1616
Dutch botanist and physician Lobelius (Mathias de l'Obel) lived.

1653
Nicholas Culpeper, wrote *The English Physician*.

1785
English doctor, William Withering, linked foxglove with heart disorders.

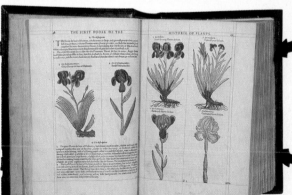

1597 The famous English herbalist, John Gerard, wrote *The Great Herball* or *Generall Historie of Plantes* (above).

1864
The National Institute of Medical Herbalists is founded in Britain.

Aloe vera

1950
Aloe vera gained popular fame as a treatment for radiation burns.

15th century
Spice routes opened up between Europe and the Middle East. Introduction of senna, cardamom, turmeric, ginger, nutmeg and cinnamon into Europe.

1624–89
Thomas Sydenham, the English physician, standardised the formula of laudanum, based on the opium poppy and modern herbalism begins.

1990
A compound from the Pacific yew – taxol – was researched as a possible cancer treatment.

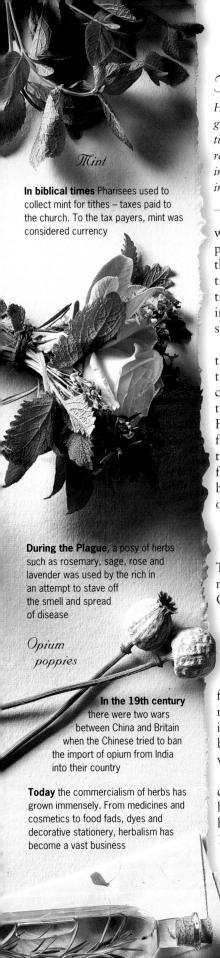

Mint

In biblical times Pharisees used to collect mint for tithes – taxes paid to the church. To the tax payers, mint was considered currency

During the Plague, a posy of herbs such as rosemary, sage, rose and lavender was used by the rich in an attempt to stave off the smell and spread of disease

Opium poppies

In the 19th century there were two wars between China and Britain when the Chinese tried to ban the import of opium from India into their country

Today the commercialism of herbs has grown immensely. From medicines and cosmetics to food fads, dyes and decorative stationery, herbalism has become a vast business

The Currency of Herbs

Herbs have played such an important part in the growth of so many societies that they have at times been used as currency and come to represent wealth and social position. The importance of the herb and spice trade has led to international unrest and even war.

with that of priest. In Siberia, Lapland and parts of North America and in West Africa, the priest or shaman would induce a state of trance in himself and his patients, sometimes with the aid of hallucinogenic plants, in order to commune with the spirit of the sick person.

The apothecaries and physicians among the European settlers in North America took their own drugs with them and were contemptuous of the idea that they had anything to learn from the Native Americans. Fortunately, unlettered people living on the frontier were not so dismissive. Thus it is that European herbalists learnt of the benefits of squaw vine, false indigo, blue and black cohosh roots, goldenseal and many other plants from North America.

FROM CULPEPER TO THE MODERN DAY

The modern approach to herbal remedies may be seen as beginning with Nicholas Culpeper. He advocated the use of natural local flora to cure ills and to help the poor to avoid the expensive foreign herbs that many doctors prescribed.

His books brought herbal remedies into many people's homes, and popular opinion forced acceptance of indigenous herbal remedies. This helped to push out the growing numbers of herbal quacks and mountebanks who plied their generally worthless wares around the countryside.

The demands for acceptable herbal remedies that actually worked to combat disease led to greater interest and investment in herbalism and medicine in the 18th and 19th centuries. The growth of patent medicines and scientific testing for active herbal and natural ingredients led to great leaps in the understanding of therapeutic herbal preparations.

Herbalism itself began to branch into diverse disciplines such as homeopathy, Bach flower remedies and, by the early 20th century, aromatherapy.

During the 20th century the growth of scientific research has further exposed the therapeutic power of plant-based remedies, and the development of transport and storage has meant that the scope for gathering herbs has extended worldwide.

Reassessing herbalism and superstition

There has been a long tradition linking herbal remedies and preparations with magic, witchcraft and superstition. It is often assumed, however, that if a plant is associated with a superstition, any claimed medicinal use of the plant must be false.

Superstitious fallacies arise when a culture believes in its traditions and practices, even when the belief contradicts personal experience. In the Middle Ages in northern Europe, medical practice was entrenched in superstition and the majority of people were actively discouraged from using and trusting their own observation. Early civilisations rarely had the luxury of superstitious fallacy, however, without personal or tribal experience of poisonous plants they could easily die if they ceased to trust their senses. Therefore, although some herbal remedies may be based purely on superstition, we must not dismiss all herbal remedies as ancient superstitious foolishness.

DOCTRINE OF SIGNATURES

The medieval belief that plants look like the organs or illnesses that they can cure was known as the doctrine of signatures. Whether Nature somehow developed a system of signs as to the medicinal value of plants is open to conjecture. Nevertheless, many coincidences between plant shape and action are borne out by scientific fact. Yellow plants, for example, were thought to be effective treatment for jaundice. Science has since proved that some plants with yellow latex, such as greater celandine, have powerful effects upon the smooth muscle of the bile duct taking bile from the liver and relieving jaundice. Similarly, the white flowers of white deadnettle were used to treat the white discharge of thrush. We now know that they do ease thrush.

STUDIES OF AGE-OLD REMEDIES

Despite a wealth of historical knowledge it is only in the last century or so that traditional herbal remedies have been the subject of serious scientific study.

The 19th century was the great age of the patent medicine. Tinctures, cordials and electuaries – medicinal powders mixed with honey or other sweeteners – were peddled by travelling quacks and also promoted by the simultaneous rise of advertising and retail pharmacies. Once plants were shown to have real value, many suffered the fate of becoming known as a panacea. The word literally means 'a cure for all things' and many valuable plants bear this optimistic hope among their common names.

Such widespread and unrealistic expectations, however, led inevitably to disappointment and to the steady and eventual decline of herbal remedies, many of which have since been scientifically proven to have valid medicinal applications.

Increasingly in recent years, scientific research into herbal remedies has focused on popular traditional remedies. Many clinical studies of the healing properties of some of the earliest medicinal herbs used have given excellent results. Amongst the many herbs subjected to clinical study three have emerged of particular interest: barberry, feverfew and valerian.

Barberry *(Berberis vulgaris)*

A densely branched shrub with spines and yellow wood, barberry bears bright red oblong-shaped berries in autumn. The bark of the root is considered by herbalists to be a highly effective remedy for gall-bladder disease. In the Middle Ages, the doctrine of signatures recommended barberry flowers as a treatment for jaundice. It has to be

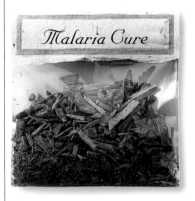

BARBERRY
The ancient Egyptians used barberry as a cure for fevers – pre-empting the current interest in the plant to relieve malaria, a disease characterised by its high fevers.

THE SEARCH FOR A CURE-ALL

Between the 18th and early 20th centuries there grew a widespread fashion for quacks – unqualified medical practitioners – to travel the countryside selling often worthless concoctions as restoratives and panaceas. This led to a growing distrust of herbal and natural cures and may have set back the acceptance of herbal remedies for many years. Fortunately, modern research has brought traditional herbal remedies to the fore again.

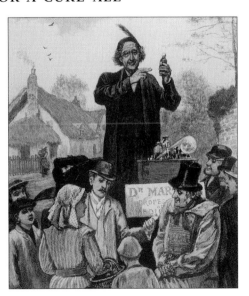

MOUNTEBANKS
The growth of the market for miracle cures in Europe gave rise to mountebanks – travelling 'quacks' who would address their audience from a raised platform or grassy bank.

administered with great care, for adverse reactions, usually diarrhoea, are not uncommon, especially in the elderly. Barberry must at all costs be avoided during pregnancy because it acts as a uterine stimulant and may lead to miscarriage, although it can in no way be considered a safe method of termination for a pregnancy. The ripe fruit, rich in vitamin C, is made into jelly; the green fruit may be pickled and used like capers, but it is best to try to exclude the stones. The wood is used for toothpicks.

The most recent pharmaceutical interest in barberry has focused on its action against disease-causing protozoa. These are microscopic organisms that are carried in the blood of larger insects, such as mosquitos, and which cause diseases like malaria.

It has also been scientifically demonstrated that barberry is toxic to the causative organism in Leishmaniasis, a tropical skin disease transmitted by sandflies which is notoriously resistant to conventional medical treatment and therefore in desperate need of another form of cure.

Feverfew *(Tanacetum parthenium)*

This is a bitter herb with a strong smell like camphor. It was traditionally employed as a digestive tonic and mild sedative and is used in France as an infusion for insomnia. Since the 1970s, scientific and clinical studies have shown that feverfew's other folk reputation as a gentle treatment for migraine is also well justified.

The medicinal use of feverfew leaves was first recorded in Greece as a remedy for young women (parthenos) and the various disorders to which they are susceptible. This may well be the reason why it was so highly favoured by herbalists during the Renaissance and used as a treatment for painful menstruation: Culpeper even recommends feverfew being applied as a warm poultice 'to the privy parts' to relieve discomfort.

An earlier application, however, was as a remedy for migraine, an affliction more commonly seen in women than men which often makes its first appearance at puberty.

In recent years, scientists have become more interested in the potential application of feverfew as a treatment for arthritis. Studies have examined the effect that extracts of feverfew have upon the activity of blood platelets and upon certain changes in human membranes. These changes, which are almost certainly involved in the onset of migraine, may also be related to the development of arthritis.

Feverfew can cause contact dermatitis in susceptible individuals and eating the fresh young leaves, the traditional method of taking the herb, caused mouth ulcers in 11.3 per cent of patients who took part in a clinical trial; digestive disturbances (but with no evidence of peptic ulceration) were reported by a further 6.5 per cent. Nonetheless, even with these possible allergic reactions, the outlook for feverfew as a major help in the battle against arthritis is very positive.

Valerian *(Valeriana officinalis)*

The first mention of valerian as medicine seems to have come from the plant list of Isaac Judaeus, physician to the rulers of Qairawan, part of the great Islamic culture of North Africa in the 9th century. In the later Middle Ages, it came to be valued as a panacea both north and south of the Alps.

The botanist Fabio Colonna, who was born in Naples in 1567, tried to overcome his epilepsy with plant medicines and, following the advice of Dioscorides, claims to have been cured by valerian. A number of other species from around the world have similar reputations; marsh valerian was used by the Menomini peoples of central North America, and there is a valerian in the Indian Pharmacopoeia.

Valerian root is an extremely effective calming and relaxing remedy, especially for people suffering from anxiety, restlessness or stress-related insomnia. Its action is complex and it is reported to have an enhancing, almost stimulating edge to the sedative properties for which it is so valued.

A great deal of research has been conducted into the pharmacology of the plant constituents and the scientific findings tend to confirm the view that a complex interaction of active substances is responsible for the effects rather than a single class of compounds. These findings may explain the fact that valerian is unique in its effects, and that the whole plant is needed to achieve them.

Feverfew and Valerian Tea
to relieve headaches

2 tbsp dried, chopped valerian root
2 tbsp dried feverfew
2 tbsp dried camomile flowers

■ Mix the three herbs together in an airtight tin and shake to distribute them evenly.
■ To make up the tea, infuse 1 tsp of the mix in a cup of boiling water for 5 minutes.
■ Take up to three times a day. Do not take for more than two to three weeks without a break.

HERBS AND PHARMACEUTICALS

Although many drugs are based on extracts from plants, there are significant differences in the way herbalists and pharmacists view their medicinal applications.

In the first half of the 19th century, technological improvements in the microscope contributed to a number of breakthroughs in the study of medicinal plants. Quinine, for instance, was extracted from the bark of the South American cinchona tree in 1820 by the French pharmacists Jean-Baptiste Caventou and Pierre-Joseph Pelletier, who also discovered caffeine in coffee. Quinine remained the principal treatment for malaria until quite recently. Just 15 years earlier in Germany, the apothecary Freidrich Sertürner had isolated morphine from the opium poppy. Opium was then probably the most widely used painkiller and was shown to yield codeine, but its addictive nature was not fully appreciated.

Some of the other active plant-elements found at that time are still prescribed today as individual drugs – digoxin, for example, for its stimulating effect upon the failing heart, atropine for its antispasmodic effect upon smooth muscle in the eye, salivary glands and the bowel, and colchicine for the treatment of acute episodes of gout. Others, like strychnine, were not developed because they proved too toxic for general human use.

In North America, Samuel Thomson (1769–1843) developed herbal medicines based on traditional Native American herbs. His simplistic approach to the value of these herbs, however, was dismissed by the American doctor, Wooster Beech, in the 1930s. Beech looked closely at Thomson's herbal remedies and conventional treatments and combined them to utilise the best of both. This led to greater acceptance of herbal remedies by conventional medics.

As research progressed, the modern pharmaceutical industry was born. From the outset, herbs were recognised as having
continued on page 30

Pharmacognosy

The term pharmacognosy was coined by a chemist in 1815. Unlike pharmacology, which is the study of the actions and uses of drugs, pharmacognosy – literal meaning 'to acquire knowledge of drugs' – refers to the scientific analysis and identification of medicinal plants. The rise of pharmaceutical chemistry in the 19th century, along with developments in botanical science, led scientists to examine plant medicines in a systematic way. The isolation of chemical substances from plants showed that there was more to plant matter than met the eye: it became clear that there is enormous variation in the substances produced by different parts of a herb and by different herbs.

MALARIA

Carried and spread by the bite of a mosquito, malaria is a very serious disease that affects over 300 million people worldwide every year. The severity of the attacks and symptoms varies depending on the type of mosquito that infects the bloodstream.

Minute parasites called protozoa infect red blood cells. Symptoms appear when infected red blood cells rupture and release more protozoa into the bloodstream. Some herbs have an antiprotozoal action – toxic to the malaria-causing protozoa – and can therefore relieve malaria.

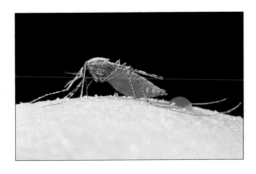

ANOPHELES MOSQUITO
The female mosquito injects protozoa into the bloodstream as she feeds. There are four types of protozoa, known as plasmodia, that can cause malaria in humans.

The Pharmacognosist

Importers and retailers of medicinal plants, as well as herbs and spices for food flavourings, need to know that what they are buying is authentic and uncontaminated. In order to do this, they employ the services of a pharmacognosist.

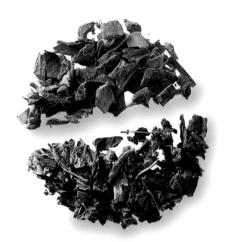

ASPIRIN AND SALICIN
The salicin found in willow and meadowsweet, above, was the forerunner of modern aspirin. Research into salicin's analgesic action led to vast improvements in modern pharmaceutical pain relievers.

Since the 1940s the dominance of chemical medicine and the routine use of antibiotics in conventional medical treatment has meant that pharmacists have had little use of pharmacognosy and its place on the university syllabus for pharmacy has declined. Conversely, in Britain, contemporary herbalists who take a degree in Herbal Medicine find that pharmacognosy is an important part of their training because it ensures that they have a thorough knowledge of the plants and plant extracts that they are using.

What qualifications are needed and where do they train?
Pharmacognosists will have a first degree in pharmacy from a university or school of pharmacy. Having trained along with pharmacists, they will be qualified to work as dispensing chemists. If they knew in advance that they wanted to become pharmacognosists, students may have chosen an establishment that still offers courses in this particular speciality. Modern high-street chemists have little need for the skills of the pharmacognosist, and so most degree courses in pharmacy have dispensed with it.

Where do they work?
Until recently, pharmacognosists tended to work in the few schools of pharmacy that continued to teach the subject. However, as more drug companies are investigating plants for use in medicine, the skills of the pharmacognosist are once more in demand. Drug companies do not wish to use plants directly, but are interested in some of the compounds that they contain. They will research the chemical to see if it can be used directly, or as a starter for a similar but entirely new compound. Salicin, for example, found in meadowsweet and willow was the raw material for acetysalicylic acid (aspirin) which does not occur naturally.

The work of other research institutes, such as the Jodrell Laboratory at Kew, depends upon the combined efforts of plant scientists and pharmacognosists.

THE JODRELL LABORATORY AT KEW

The original Jodrell Laboratory at The Royal Botanic Gardens, Kew, in London was established in 1876 to study and analyse the famous collection of flora collected by the staff of the botanic gardens. This original building, with only four rooms allotted to research, was in use until 1965 when it was demolished to make way for a newer, larger laboratory.

This current laboratory is nearly ten times the size of its predecessor and has room for 60 staff. Current work in progress is furthering understanding about new natural medicines from plants, seed conservation and projects such as improving fuelwoods for the developing world. The laboratory focuses on research, conservation and furthering the scientific and medical knowledge about plants from all over the world.

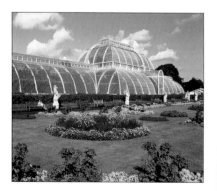

KEW GARDENS
The beautiful gardens at Kew are home to a vast collection of plants and herbs from around the world and therefore make an ideal setting for one of the foremost centres for pharmacognosy in the world.

Do pharmacognosists treat the public with medicinal plants?

No. Although pharmacognosists possess an enormous amount of knowledge of plants, their work is in research and teaching rather than practising medicine. Some dispensing pharmacists, depending upon where they were trained, will have a grounding in pharmacognosy, especially in France, Germany and south-eastern Europe where herbs are sold over the counter, but that will not be their main function. Pharmacognosy is concerned with the herb at every stage – from collection, drying, storing and shipping of plants through to the wholesale and even retail stage, but not working with the end consumer. However, if a complaint is made about a plant product, it may be sent to a pharmacognosist for analysis.

If you wanted to authenticate a one-off sample of a herbal 'drug', you could send it to a school of pharmacy that had a pharmacognosy department. Exporters and importers of 'crude drugs' may employ a full-time pharmacognosist as part of their quality control, depending upon the size of the business.

How are herbs analysed?

The first part of the analysis requires a deep understanding of plant morphology: the detailed shape and structure of plant tissues. By testing first by eye, then by smell and taste and then with a microscope, the content of the material can be clearly established. The next stage is to discover whether the material has been mixed with some other inert plant matter, or with any non-plant substance, either by carelessness, accident or fraudulent design.

PRACTICAL PHARMACOGNOSY
A pharmacognosist must unearth the secrets of a plant at its most fundamental levels. To understand a plant's make-up, a pharmacognosist will dissect and distil the plant until its contents are distinguishable from one another.

After the biological analysis of the plant, the pharmacognosist analyses its chemistry. The pharmacognosist has to establish whether the desired active constituents from the plant are actually present in the required amounts and have not been lost through poor harvesting or drying. Chemical tests will also check for adulteration with inorganic fillers and whether the herb is free from toxic materials such as heavy metals.

What are the tools of the trade?

Apart from the skills and 'nose' of all detectives, the pharmacognosist depends primarily upon the microscope for authentication of the plant material. However for chemical analysis, plant constituents are first extracted by the application of a series of chemical solvents, then separated by well-established laboratory techniques such as fractional distillation and crystallisation. In the last 50 years, the instrumentation and technique known as chromatography has allowed the pharmacognosist to identify minute amounts of organic molecules which before would have remained undetected, and to separate complex mixtures with a subtlety previously unimaginable. To clarify the structures of natural compounds, the professional will rely upon the specialised equipment and techniques of the analytical chemist. Indeed, many tools and methods of elucidation, such as spectroscopy, X-ray crystallography and magnetic resonance, are now commonplace tools in most branches of technical science, from astronomy to medicine.

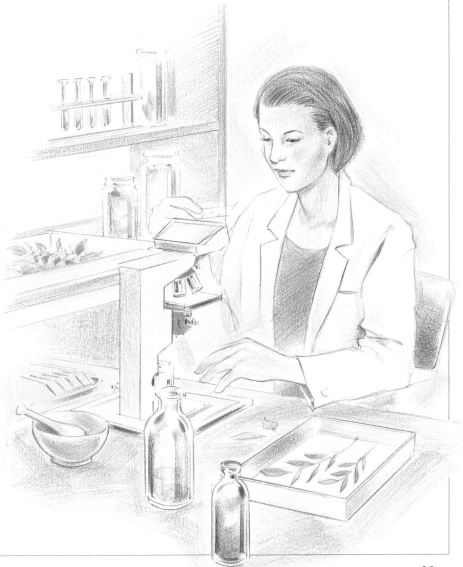

NATURAL HEALING

There is a long healing tradition involving natural products like mould and spiders' webs, lichens and mosses to treat wounds and speed healing. They are usually applied directly to the skin and their proven effectiveness no doubt comes from their natural antibiotic properties.

SPHAGNUM MOSS
The British government used tons of sphagnum moss as surgical dressing, placed directly on to wounds, towards the end of the First World War when the demand for cotton bandages could not be met. Fortunately, this folk remedy had not faded from memory. It is still used in rural areas.

important healing properties, and yet a major divide arose between the pharmaceutical industry and herbalists.

Why doctors prefer drugs and herbalists prefer herbs

The extraction of single substances from plants enabled chemists to purify and standardise remedial drugs. Pharmacists work on the basic assumption that if a drug can be shown to produce a physiological effect on a number of people, such as diminishing pain, or altering heart beat, muscle tone or mood, then it will have more or less the same effect on all people. Of course, individual adjustments can be made, but on the whole the drug is not tailored for the individual but for the condition.

Herbalists, in contrast, emphasise that there is no such thing as a 'standard' patient and place the emphasis on the person to be treated. A herbal prescription is selected by matching qualities of plants with the individual patient. This allows for minute adjustments of dosage. Only rarely will two patients receive exactly the same treatment for the same ailment.

While pharmacists generally prescribe a very precise dosage of a single powerful substance, herbalists work with a plant that may contain several hundred different substances. As well as the so-called 'active constituents' which have a definite and repeatable action on the body, as drugs do, the material may contain large amounts of relatively inert material, such as gums, mucilages, chlorophyll or fibre. Some of this material may have a 'ballast' effect and alter absorption of the active ingredients. These substances may also influence distribution to the tissues and the action there – sometimes holding back a drastic effect or amplifying an otherwise weak effect. Indeed, many of a herb's 'impurities' may in fact promote its therapeutic effects.

Is one person's heartburn the same as another's?

If a patient suffers from heartburn and the doctor considers that the patient is secreting too much acid from the stomach and not enough protective mucus, a drug which helps

protect the stomach and is also antacid may be prescribed. As soon as use of the drug is discontinued, however, it is quite likely that the condition will recur.

If the same patient consulted a herbalist, the idea behind the treatment might not seem that different. Plants which modify gastric secretion will be given along with others to protect the stomach lining. However, the object behind the treatment will be to resolve the condition so that it does not recur. Herbalists consider that the complexity of the plant constituents have a much broader action and it is not necessary to suppress the stomach acid, which is there for the purpose of properly digesting our food after all. Quite apart from the relative merits of one treatment regime over another, the herbalist will devote a considerable amount of time to dietary and lifestyle influences and perhaps recommend permanent changes and even auxiliary treatments, such as massage or relaxation exercises.

In spite of the contrast between these approaches, a good number of herbal extracts have been standardised for a particular constituent and are sold in chemists as over-the-counter medicines. In Germany, France and parts of Eastern Europe, doctors frequently prescribe such herbal preparations. The popularity of their use is ascribed to their low toxicity and the low incidence of unwanted 'side effects'.

Germany currently boasts the world's largest market for herbal remedies. In 1995, figures for Germany show that standardised extracts of *Ginkgo biloba* and *Hypericum perforatum* (St John's wort) outsold conventional drug equivalents. Recent research has shown that hypericum is at least as effective in the treatment of depression as drug therapy, without the troubling side effects.

CHAPTER 2

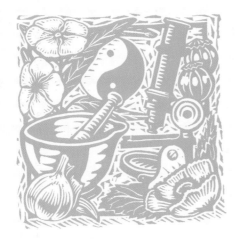

CURRENT USE OF HERBS

---

*Applications of herbal remedies are found in every
culture in the world and there are many therapies
which make use of plants to heal and relieve illness.
These include well-known therapies such as
homeopathy and Bach flower remedies, as well as
more exotic herbal treatments from as far afield as
Tibet, Pakistan and Africa.*

HERBS IN VARIOUS THERAPIES

Everywhere in the world there is some form of folk medicine involving plants. Practice varies from purely domestic use to countries with a formal system of herbal medicine.

NATURAL MEDICINE AROUND THE WORLD
From every continent the knowledge and use of herbal medicine has grown and developed. Almost all societies have offered new approaches and healing remedies to modern herbalism and one of the major challenges facing medical herbalists is to keep traditional remedies alive while furthering accurate scientific research.

There are clearly defined differences between continents and countries in the uses and approaches to herbal medicine. Western herbalism – originating in ancient Egypt, Mesopotamia, Persia and Greece – has evolved and developed in Europe since the Renaissance. Today it is widely practised in Europe, Australia, and New Zealand and is also popular in Canada and the USA.

Chinese herbalism has an unbroken tradition stretching back to ancient times. It has achieved worldwide renown and is now practised in many countries beyond its homeland. Other approaches less well known in the West are also widely prevalent in some parts of the world. Despite certain similarities in the therapeutic approaches, there are fundamental differences that separate the various systems of medicine from one another.

HERBS IN THE WESTERN WORLD
The use of plants as medicines in the West declined for decades as the popularity of chemical drugs grew. Recently, however, more people are turning to natural remedies and a more holistic approach to health.

Western herbalism
Western herbalism developed from ancient ideas about the four fluids or humours which were believed to govern illness. Today, the concept is of historical interest only, but herbalists are reluctant to simply discard some of the clinical observations

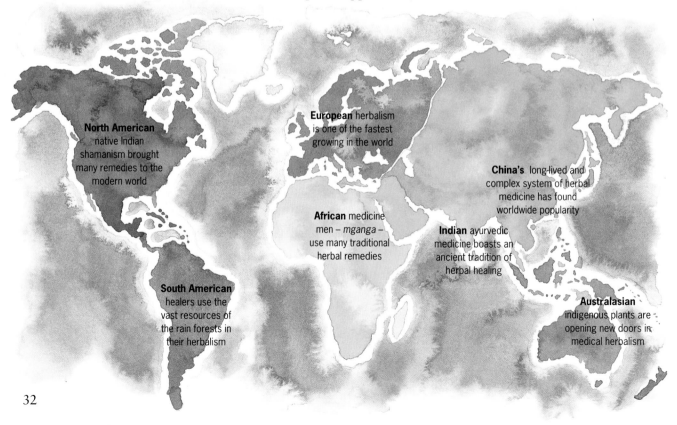

North American native Indian shamanism brought many remedies to the modern world

European herbalism is one of the fastest growing in the world

China's long-lived and complex system of herbal medicine has found worldwide popularity

African medicine men – *mganga* – use many traditional herbal remedies

Indian ayurvedic medicine boasts an ancient tradition of herbal healing

South American healers use the vast resources of the rain forests in their herbalism

Australasian indigenous plants are opening new doors in medical herbalism

embedded in these pre-scientific ideas. Herbalists who train in western Europe receive a scientific education which applies principles of modern biology both to medicinal plants and to the health of the patients. Nonetheless, many traditional folklore remedies have proven healing properties and retain a place in modern herbalism.

In the UK there are currently over 400 registered herbalists, but mainstream medicine seems unwilling to accept the claims of herbalism, despite the growing interest from the general public. This situation may be exacerbated by the fact that, although a GP can refer a patient to a herbalist, in order to prescribe herbal remedies the GP must take an exam in herbalism. This is unlikely to be practical, even for the most enlightened GPs. Further, herbs are regulated either as foods or as patented medicines, but a vast number of therapeutic herbal doses fall into neither of these categories, and therefore remain outside strict regulation. This may make some doctors and prospective patients less confident in the practice of herbal medicine and the remedies prescribed.

In Australia, officials have reacted to this problem by setting up a new area of regulation that deals purely with herbs in their own right. This, in turn, gives greater authority to the herbalist whose patients can feel confident in the remedies.

In Germany, conventional medical practitioners are far more ready to accept that herbalism has a rightful place in mainstream medicine. Many German doctors prescribe herbal remedies and there is a growing belief that the natural healing properties of herbs may, in some cases, be more therapeutic than conventional drug treatment.

Aromatherapy

This is a form of medicine which depends entirely upon plants but does not use whole plant tissue, only the volatile oil obtained from it. They are often known as 'essential oils' because they were thought to contain the 'essence' of a plant.

As aromatic oils are derived from medicinal plants, herbalists tend to view aromatherapy as a branch of herbal medicine. In general they prefer to use the whole plant for gentle efficacy and safety, but they do use oils in certain circumstances. The concentrated power and portability of oils makes them useful for first aid.

USING ESSENTIAL OILS SAFELY

All essential oils should be used in half doses during pregnancy. Basil, clove, cinnamon, fennel, hyssop, marjoram, myrrh, peppermint, rosemary, sage and thyme oils should be avoided altogether at this time because they have stimulating and emmenagogue actions which may induce miscarriage. Essential oils are highly concentrated and must be used with caution. If you are in any doubt, consult a qualified professional before using oils.

▶ During a massage, essential oils are never applied neat to the skin but must be blended with a carrier oil. For the minimum effective dose add one part of your chosen essential oil to 100 parts carrier oil, such as grapeseed or almond oil. For the maximum dose, add one part essential oil to 50 parts carrier oil. Never exceed the maximum dose and check oils for any specific contraindications.

▶ Only lavender and tea tree oils are safe for use in their undiluted states, but should only be used in small amounts.

▶ No other oil should be used in its undiluted state.

▶ Avoid getting essential oils in your eyes – they can cause permanent damage. Keep your eyes closed during inhalations.

▶ Never leave children unattended with essential oils.

▶ Never take essential oils internally.

▶ Never use more than 10 drops of essential oil in the bath.

▶ Never use higher than 2.5% dilution of essential oils in bath water.

Homeopathy

Practitioners of homeopathy believe in two important principles which determine the medication. The first is summed up in the phrase that 'like cures like'. This means that a substance that causes the symptoms of an illness can be administered to cure a patient suffering from that illness. The second is

continued on page 36

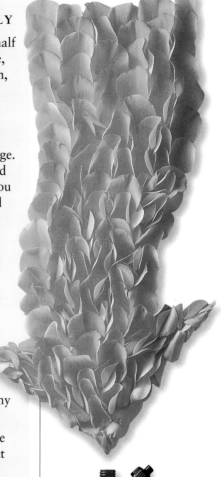

ESSENTIAL OILS
Essential oils extracted from petals are many times more expensive than those taken from other plant parts because petals yield very little of their natural oil. Rose oil, which cannot be synthetically reproduced, is particularly expensive: rose petals yield only 0.02% of their oil through steam distillation and it takes 100 kg (240 lb) of rose petals to extract just 50 g (1¾ oz)of the essential oil. Extraction by solvent, rather than steam, yields more oil, but of a lower quality.

The Aromatherapist

Many people visit aromatherapists to help them to unwind and relax. The use of aromatic oils brings a deeper relaxation than just massage and may benefit the general physical and mental well-being of the patient.

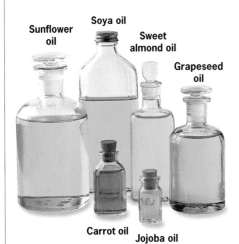

Sunflower oil

Soya oil

Sweet almond oil

Grapeseed oil

Carrot oil   Jojoba oil

OILS AND CARRIER OILS
Essential oils must be diluted in a 'base' or 'carrier' oil before use. Soya, sunflower, grapeseed and sweet almond oils make good carrier oils for body massage. For use on the face, and especially for people with sensitive skin, carrot or jojoba oils are more suitable, although they are also more expensive.

Aromatherapy is gaining widespread acceptance in the UK for its therapeutic effects, both from individuals hoping to relieve specific problems to conventional hospitals introducing aromatherapy for their patients. Indeed, many patients have been found to recover faster after aromatherapy sessions.

What training is involved in aromatherapy?
For the interested amateur, intensive courses are available that last one or two weekends or longer courses of six to ten weeks may be offered,

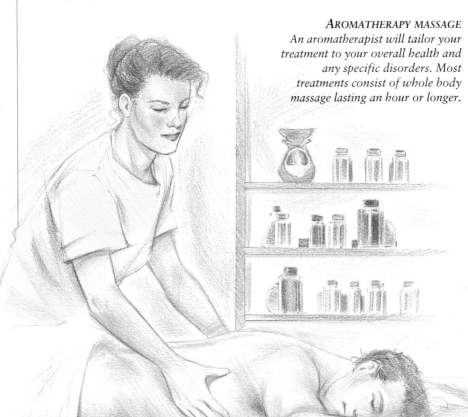

*AROMATHERAPY MASSAGE
An aromatherapist will tailor your treatment to your overall health and any specific disorders. Most treatments consist of whole body massage lasting an hour or longer.*

often by local authorities and adult education centres. For those who wish to practise professionally, a certificated course which lasts from six months to a year is a more responsible option. Shorter, intensive courses are available at some centres for nurses and other health-care professionals who already have a medical or paramedical background.

In most countries (France being a notable exception) aromatherapy is not practised by doctors and would not be seen as a medical treatment unless given by a qualified medical herbalist or other professional with medical training.

A good indication of the suitability and expertise of a therapist can be gleaned from the length of time they have been in practice, the length of their training and whether or not they are fully insured.

What is a treatment like?
Before treatment the aromatherapist will ask questions about recent health problems, allergies and emotional states. You will then remove your clothes, depending on the extent of the massage required. Because not every part of the body can be massaged at once, even for a full body massage, those parts not being treated will remain covered.

The therapist will incorporate essential oils into the carrier oil, which may in fact be a good cooking oil, such as sunflower or soya.

Typically, however, a lighter oil such as grapeseed is used because it leaves the patient feeling less oily. The traditional choice is almond oil of pharmaceutical grade, but some therapists prefer to use a rich nutritious oil, such as avocado, hazelnut or wheatgerm.

What effects do aromatic oils have?
Smells can evoke memories and affect emotions, especially if they are inhaled when the body and mind are relaxed. Most people like the aroma of freshly cut hay, flowers, woodland and spices, but there are great differences in preferences even with smells that are generally considered agreeable – a pleasant smell for one person may be repulsive to another.

It is therefore important to make a distinction between the effect of perfumes and pleasant smells, which are fleeting and not experienced in a therapeutic context, and the influence of aromatic oils of plants. Aromatic oils have an added effect on the body when the patient inhales the aroma during treatment.

Some aromatherapists believe that plant oils absorbed through the skin during massage provoke beneficial hormonal and emotional responses.

How are the oils selected?
There are about 40 plant oils currently in common use, chosen from the many hundreds in nature, and most therapists would keep between one and two dozen of these in stock. The oils may be classified according to their effects upon the body – for example, whether they are relaxing, stimulating or uplifting – and the nature of the aroma, such as woody, herbaceous or fruity.

The therapist will choose according to the patient's physical and emotional state. The therapist will monitor the patient's reactions to the treatment throughout.

The effect of an oil and its aroma type can vary considerably depending, like a wine, upon the soil on which it was grown and the season in which it was harvested. Some lavenders can produce an oil that is almost citrus in aroma, which can be invigorating, while other

lavender oils resemble the aroma of pine and have the effect of relaxing and lowering any levels of anxiety. Any oil made from basil is uplifting with a warm and spicy aroma, with hints of camphor and fruit, while fennel oil stimulates and refreshes and also has a warm, yet fruity aroma. An aromatherapist will have a good knowledge of the effects of the oils they recommend.

Are there any side effects?
It is fairly common for clients to become so relaxed they fall asleep during treatment. If this happens it is important that they are allowed adequate time to 'come to', to get up slowly and dress unhurriedly. If a deeply relaxed state has been induced it may not be safe for the patient to drive or operate machinery until they are fully awake. But it should be emphasised that the person has not been 'drugged' in any way: judgement is often very clear and enhanced. People with very sensitive skin may develop a slight irritation if the blend of oil is strong, but this will show immediately and can be adjusted by the therapist.

Origins

In the 1920s, the French chemist Rene Gattefossé's work with plant oils inspired the French doctor, Jean Valnet. Valnet used the oils on wounds in the Second World War and his book *Aromathérapie* in 1964 made such treatment popular with the general public.

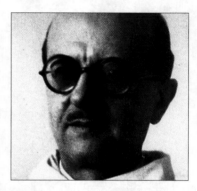

RENE GATTEFOSSÉ
When Gattefossé badly burned his arm in a laboratory accident, he plunged it into a vat of lavender oil. The burn healed so quickly and well that he became intrigued by the healing effects of plant oils.

WHAT YOU CAN DO AT HOME

Adding drops of an oil such as lavender to your bath can enhance its relaxing effects. However, it is important to remember that the oils are very concentrated and that less is more. Quite apart from being toxic, if the amount added is excessive, the oil can have the opposite to its intended effect, stimulating and irritating the nerves rather than relaxing them. It is always crucial, therefore, to check the dosage on the bottle and never exceed it.

Aromatherapy oils are effective as inhalants for upper respiratory infections in both children and adults. Care must be taken, however, to measure the number of drops used and monitor the length of time of exposure, otherwise the delicate nasal lining may become damaged.

BATH BENEFITS
Oils should be added to bath water while the taps are running. Never use more than ten drops of oil in a bath.

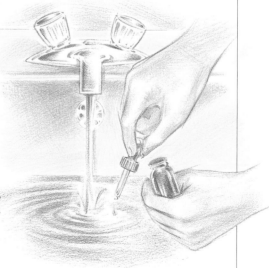

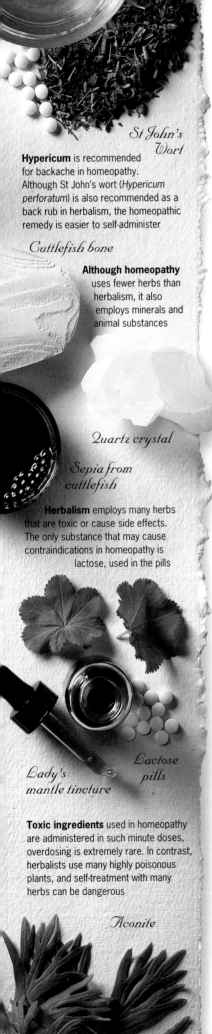

Hypericum is recommended for backache in homeopathy. Although St John's wort (*Hypericum perforatum*) is also recommended as a back rub in herbalism, the homeopathic remedy is easier to self-administer

St John's Wort

Cuttlefish bone

Although homeopathy uses fewer herbs than herbalism, it also employs minerals and animal substances

Quartz crystal

Sepia from cuttlefish

Herbalism employs many herbs that are toxic or cause side effects. The only substance that may cause contraindications in homeopathy is lactose, used in the pills

Lady's mantle tincture

Lactose pills

Toxic ingredients used in homeopathy are administered in such minute doses, overdosing is extremely rare. In contrast, herbalists use many highly poisonous plants, and self-treatment with many herbs can be dangerous

Aconite

Why Use Homeopathy?

Many of the herbs used in homeopathy are toxic yet, in correct doses, homeopathic pills have no contraindications, except for people who are lactose intolerant and would have to use homeopathic tinctures instead. They can therefore be safely and easily self-administered over long periods of time.

that the smaller the dose the more effective the treatment; if the active ingredient in a remedy is diluted in a particular manner (see below) the therapeutic effect becomes more powerful. As the doses are infinitesimal, there is no toxic effect.

The medicinal substances of homeopathy may come from an animal, vegetable or mineral source. If the starting material is a herb, it is always used fresh and made into an alcoholic tincture – in effect, a weak herbal medicine. The homeopath proceeds to make a series of dilutions or 'potentisations', to produce medicines of the required strength. These are usually taken in the form of a white pill which is placed under the tongue.

Homeopathic treatment is often confused with herbal medicine because many homeopathic remedies are derived from plants. The distinction, however, lies in the microscopic dosages prescribed in homeopathy and the different approach to treatment. For example, homeopaths may give a minute dose of arnica for emotional shock, while herbalists would not prescribe it for internal use because it is toxic at strengths required by herbal medicine. Herbalists make an ointment of the flowerheads of arnica which can be applied to bruises, sprains, unbroken chilblains and acne.

Even more remarkable is the case of aconite – a plant so toxic that it should never be put on unbroken skin: some herbalists will not handle the fresh root unless they are wearing gloves.

By contrast, the homeopathic remedy aconite is sold over the counter for a wide range of symptoms, including sore throat, dry cough, anxiety, restlessness, fear, grief and insomnia. Also the manner in which symptoms arise are considered important by homeopaths – for instance, whether a chill followed exposure to dry, cold winds or chilly, damp weather – and can affect the recommended treatment.

Bach flower remedies

Dr Edward Bach (1886–1936) was an English bacteriologist who became convinced that personality types and emotional states contribute to illness. He believed that the 'vibrations' given off by certain plants directly influenced the human spirit. This 'attunement' led him to believe that certain plants were a direct representation of a human emotion. Mimulus, for instance, he saw as the positive response to fear and so prescribed it for those in need of courage.

Most Bach flower remedies are made by floating the freshly picked flowers on the surface of spring water in a glass bowl on a sunny morning, according to simple but exacting rules. Bach himself discovered 38 remedies. In other parts of the world, for example California, people have identified other groups of 'flower essences'.

HERBS IN OTHER CULTURES

While it is only comparatively recently that the West has rediscovered herbs, in other parts of the world herbs have maintained a central position in the treatment of illness.

Chinese medicine

Chinese herbal medicine has always had a place in Eastern therapies, but is now the focus of increased attention in the West. Unlike Western herbalism, Chinese medicine has a very firm grounding in ancient beliefs and remedies. Indeed, with its long unbroken tradition, and huge natural flora, China has the largest and most complex repertoire of medicinal herbs in the world.

The main difference between the Chinese and Western approaches lies in the philosophy behind the treatment. The Chinese believe that everything, both animate and inanimate, has a vital energy which they call *chi*. If the flow of chi through the body is disrupted, the result is illness. Chi can be disrupted by imbalances in the two ruling forces, *yin* and *yang*, and can be returned to its natural flow by treatment with herbs that counter the yin/yang imbalance. Hence, it is not so much the antiviral property of a herb that will lead to it being prescribed for a sore throat, but more the yin or yang effect the herb will have on the body's imbalance.

In this way, a Chinese herbalist does not simply treat the symptoms of an illness, but attempts to restore health to the whole of the body – a holistic approach. Nonetheless,

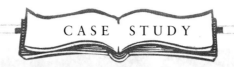

The Overstressed Woman

When a family's income or lifestyle preferences demand that both partners work, it is often still the woman who bears the brunt of the domestic load. Juggling the pressures of work, home and family can lead to undesirable stress levels for all involved, and an inequality in such pressures may lead to feelings of unfairness and anger.

Miriam is 34 and married with two children aged eight and ten. She has worked for the past five years in a supermarket and has recently decided to go to university so that she will have a greater earning capacity when the children are older. Her evening classes building up to university entrance are going well.

Her husband, Alan, is supportive and helps with the children and housework, but he has the chance of promotion at work and is having to prove himself to the company by putting in longer hours. Miriam is now finding it increasingly difficult to juggle her domestic, financial and educational commitments. She has recently begun to suffer from headaches and nausea after eating.

WHAT SHOULD MIRIAM DO?

Miriam and Alan should work out a timetable and routine for sharing all home and family duties, without adding too much strain. They also need to work out a budget for when Miriam is no longer in paid employment, so she can feel more relaxed about her future studies. A friend tells Miriam about the relief she found from herbal remedies and strongly recommends a visit to a herbalist. Miriam takes the advice and, after assessing her situation, the herbalist suggests various herbal teas and bath preparations to help Miriam to unwind and relax. These include valerian and St John's wort teas to help her to stay calm and improve concentration, and a balm bath for relaxation.

Action Plan

FAMILY
Agree what tasks need to be done each week and allow time for them to be accomplished without too much stress.

STRESS
Consult a herbalist and implement any recommendations within the daily routine.

MONEY
Work out a realistic budget and if necessary make decisions, such as to forego a holiday, to relieve the pressures of changing to a reduced income.

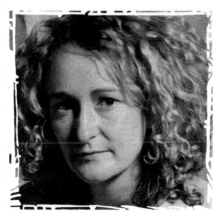

MONEY
Careful budgeting can help to relieve the pressure of changes in income.

FAMILY
An even division of family responsibilities can help both partners to feel they have time for their own needs.

STRESS
Herbal remedies can relieve tension, both physical and emotional, and aid concentration, relaxation and general well-being.

HOW THINGS TURNED OUT FOR MIRIAM

The herbs helped Miriam to relax and concentrate. She achieved good exam results and is looking forward to starting university. She is still aware of being under pressure, although she feels everybody is now sharing the load at home, and daily cups of herbal tea and a relaxing bath help her to cope. Alan got his promotion and, although he now has greater responsibility at work, he too has found the effects of the herbal remedies helpful.

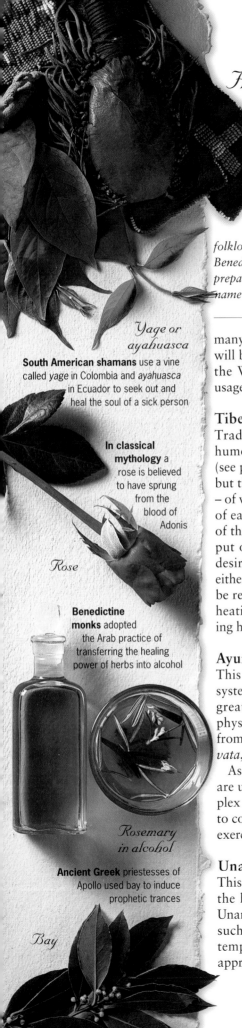

Yage or ayahuasca
South American shamans use a vine called *yage* in Colombia and *ayahuasca* in Ecuador to seek out and heal the soul of a sick person

In classical mythology a rose is believed to have sprung from the blood of Adonis

Rose

Benedictine monks adopted the Arab practice of transferring the healing power of herbs into alcohol

Rosemary in alcohol

Ancient Greek priestesses of Apollo used bay to induce prophetic trances

Bay

Herbs and Religion

Herbs have played a major role in most religions throughout the centuries. From classical traditions to African tribal ceremonies herbs have been used to alter mental states and release the user into a more spiritual awareness. Other herbs are closely linked to deities or used to symbolise them in religious tales and folklore. Some religious groups, such as the Benedictine monks, have made certain herbal preparations their own. The liqueur of the same name is still popular today.

many herbs prescribed in Chinese herbalism will be familiar to herbalists and patients in the West, even if the theory behind their usage is not.

Tibetan medicine

Traditional medicine in Tibet is essentially humoral, like ancient European herbalism (see page 32), but differs in having not four but three humours – phlegm, wind and bile – of which there are no fewer than five kinds of each mixed throughout the body. If any of the 15 varieties of the three humours are put out of balance by the three poisons – desire, hatred and confusion – the result is either a 'hot' or a 'cold' disease. Balance can be restored through herbal treatment using heating herbs for a 'cold' disease and cooling herbs for a 'hot' one.

Ayurveda

This is the name of the traditional medical system of India. Ayurvedic medicine places great emphasis on the temperament and physical constitution of the patient derived from the bodily humours or types known as *vata*, *pitta* and *kapha*.

As in Chinese medicine, medicinal plants are used with very specific, subtle and complex instructions, and attention is also given to correct breathing and improving posture, exercise and diet.

Unani

This method is practised in Pakistan where the herbal healer is known as the *hakim*. Unani has some similarities with Ayurveda, such as a concern with understanding the temperament of the sick person and with appropriate diet and lifestyle.

Unani was thought to have originated in ancient Greece and then absorbed influences from Persia, Arabia and East Africa. The extent of herbal treatment in the system is astounding. A recent study conducted by the Department of Pharmaceutical Sciences at Nottingham University investigated the use of medicinal plants by the Asian community in Britain. It found no fewer than 325 species of herbs, some European, currently being prescribed by the hakim.

East African medicine

Herbal medicine is offered on a professional basis by medicine men, especially in the Swahili-speaking region of the East African coast. The majority of these medicine men, or *mganga* as they are called, would have been apprenticed by a parent or close relative; others inherit a practice in the shape of the *mfuko*, the medicine bag. As is common in herbal treatment throughout the world, the medicine is personalised to the individual patient. Roots and barks of trees and shrubs, collected from the bush, are more often used than seeds and herbs – the ingredients are usually boiled together or soaked in water for a long time. Some mganga have also received Islamic training and may therefore also be Koran teachers, or *mwalimu*. The great advantage with both religious and traditional forms of healing, especially to the poor, is that the patients feel relaxed in the house of the mganga, and this encourages the healing process.

Central and South American medicine

The mountains, lakes, forests and even the deserts of the Americas possess an extraordinarily rich variety of flora which the many indigenous peoples have developed into a correspondingly rich practice of herbal medicine. In recent decades this medical system has been threatened, as have the plants and trees on which it depends.

The best-known areas of plant diversity and herbal healing are along the basins of two great rivers – the Amazon and the Orinoco – but a great wealth of plants is also found in the Andes in Bolivia and the Paraguayan plains. In places like Chiapas in southern Mexico, Ecuador and Guatemala, indigenous knowledge has been enhanced with European herbs and ideas, and Mediterranean medicinal herbs, such as anise, are sold alongside native medicines.

HERBAL BEAUTY PRODUCTS

From skin creams to shampoos there is a growing demand for products that contain plant extracts to improve their performance, texture or scent.

Until recently most 'herbal' beauty products contained only a small amount of botanical ingredients – usually not enough to make any difference to their cleansing performance. However, as a result of a general increased interest in 'alternative' treatments, a wider range of quality botanical products is now available.

The distinction between herbal and non-herbal products is not an easy one to draw because nearly all products contain some substance derived from a plant. Even though the fragrance of lemon-scented washing-up liquid will not have come from fresh lemons, the limonene that is used as a scent has its origin in the plant. Dyes and oils from plants have always been added for their texture, colour and, especially, their perfume but the actual cleansing properties of a product or its final texture are more usually derived from chemicals.

Products containing whole-plant extracts or which make an appeal to 'naturalness' are generally higher in price than chemical products but sell well. This is despite the fact that only a small number of plants, such as evening primrose, jojoba and witch hazel, are well enough known to the majority of consumers to sell on their own merits. Simply branding a product as 'natural' can be enough to give it instant appeal.

SKIN PREPARATIONS

Setting specific ailments aside, skin type generally falls into one of the categories in the table below. Dry skin may either lack oil, or be dehydrated through lack of moisture. 'Normal' skin has no extremes of oil or moisture, while sensitive skin is highly reactive to any number of external chemicals, as well as to insects and contact with certain plants. There are four main types of

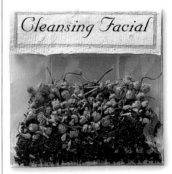

Cleansing Facial

Place 1 tbsp dried nettles and 1 tbsp dried camomile flowers in a heatproof bowl and cover with boiling water to make a cleansing facial steam for all skin types. Alternatively, select herbs to suit your skin from the chart below.

HERBS FOR YOUR SKIN TYPE

Whatever your skin type, herbs can be used to make cleansing, nourishing and healing cosmetics. Combine herbs from the different sections of the chart below to prepare a cream, lotion or cleanser for your particular skin type. See pages 75 to 80 for details on how to make the various herbal preparations.

SKIN TYPE	SYMPTOMS	HERBS RECOMMENDED	PREPARATIONS
Normal	Fine, smooth texture. No shine or flaking	Lemon verbena, nettle, rose	Cleanse with regular steaming and face packs
Oily	Heavy, unrefined texture. Shiny surface. Large pores. Blackheads	Bergamot, cypress, geranium, lavender, lemon, nettle, rosemary	Fruit or clay masks. Exfoliating scrubs. Steaming. Toning lotions
Dry	Delicate texture, prone to tightness, flaking and wrinkles	Comfrey, fennel, jasmine, neroli, lavender, rose, sandalwood	Cream-based masks and moisturisers. Aromatherapy massage with essential oils
Sensitive	Prone to redness and irritation especially after using soap or cosmetics	Comfrey, camomile, lavender, rose	Massage using jojoba oil as a carrier. Always patch test new products
Combination	Dry around cheeks, neck and eyes but oily on the 'T-zone' – nose, forehead and chin	Camomile, orange blossom, nettle, rose	Rose or orange blossom water cleansers. Massage with light carrier oil such as jojoba
Acne	Greasy, coarse skin. Spots and blackheads	Tea tree essential oil	Apply directly to affected area, 1 or 2 times a day

skin preparation, each of which takes into account and tries to balance the skin types to even out extremes of oil and dryness.

Cleansers

These remove dirt and make-up and are used in place of soap, which also removes oils from the skin. Cleansers for dry or dehydrated skin have a creamy texture with emollient properties, that is, they are soothing or softening on application. Many are designed to be removed without water.

Herbal extracts used in cleansing compounds for dry skin include cucumber, which has soothing and refreshing juices and a moisturising effect. Camomile extract is also soothing and anti-inflammatory. Essential oil of lemon balm has particularly good skin penetration and is added to high-quality cosmetic treatments for oily or acne-prone skin. Orange, lemon and bilberry extracts are valued for oily skin and for their rich content of alphahydroxy acids which astringe, cleanse and feed the skin.

Toners

Toners are meant to be refreshing and to some extent astringe or tighten the skin. Old-fashioned astringent lotions based on aluminium and zinc salts – in effect antiperspirants – have given way to a range of compounds that provide a greater degree of softness to the skin at the same time as giving tone. Herbal extracts suitable for use as toners include rose water, which has very soothing properties making it an excellent

tonic for sensitive, dry and mature skin, and sage which, with its astringent qualities, is particularly helpful for toning oily skin.

Moisturising day creams

These are formulated to hydrate the deeper layers of the skin and to provide a protective film over the surface of the skin to keep out infection and dirt. A combination of avocado and nettle make an excellent day cream as the avocado provides vitamin and oil-rich properties, while the nettle has astringent and purifying qualities.

Therapeutic skin preparations

There are many products that utilise the therapeutic effects of certain herbal extracts to repair damaged skin or relieve irritation.

Allantoin, for example, is a natural compound found in comfrey (*Symphytum officinale*). Herbalists use comfrey principally for repairing damaged connective tissue as it stimulates tissue regeneration. Allantoin is added to cleansers for its soothing properties and as an aid to retaining the elasticity of the skin, as it has an anti-wrinkle effect. Cucumber juice is also soothing and refreshing. It has a moisturising effect especially suitable for dry skin types and as a first-aid treatment for mild burns, and is one of the simplest, most accessible materials for making beauty products at home. Wheatgerm oil is an excellent source of vitamin E and is soothing and nourishing, especially to dry skin. This oil can also help to combat wrinkles and stretch marks.

COSMETICS AND IMAGERY

Like all packaging techniques, those used to sell shop-bought herbal products differ little from those used to sell any other product. Fresh, 'natural' colours and simple typefaces suggest a natural, 'unspoilt' product and the important herbal extract may appear large on the label – even though only tiny amounts may be present. If possible, buy herbal products from established and reputable suppliers or make your own.

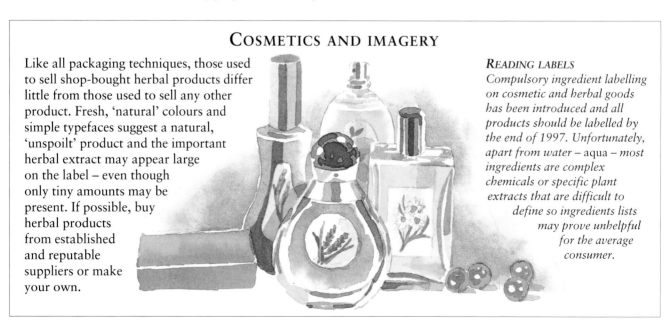

READING LABELS
Compulsory ingredient labelling on cosmetic and herbal goods has been introduced and all products should be labelled by the end of 1997. Unfortunately, apart from water – aqua – most ingredients are complex chemicals or specific plant extracts that are difficult to define so ingredients lists may prove unhelpful for the average consumer.

Herbal Face Packs

A daily facial care programme is essential for keeping your skin both healthy and clean. The further application of an occasional face pack can only enhance your complexion.

A herbal face pack, dependent upon its composition, may soften, cleanse, astringe, produce perspiration or stimulate and refresh the skin and can be tailored to suit any skin type.

The packs you use and the frequency with which you use them will depend upon your skin type, your age and whether you suffer from any skin problems.

Face packs for professional use are usually made from wax, gel or mucilage (often containing gelatin, glycerine and gums from plants). However, they may also be based on egg white (albuminous) or a milk protein, casein. In some cases they may be based on high-quality clays, earth or volcanic ash. These are described as argillaceous.

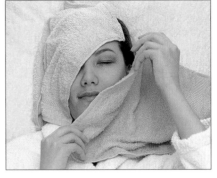

PREPARING YOUR SKIN
Add 2 drops of essential oil to a basin of hot water and soak two facecloths in it. Cover your face with the facecloths and leave until the cloths cool.

MASK FOR OILY SKIN

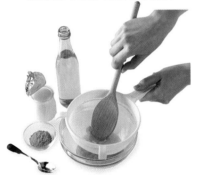

1 *Force the flesh of half a ripe papaya through a sieve into a clean bowl. Mix in 1 tbsp fuller's earth powder and 1 tbsp natural yoghurt. Add 1 tbsp of orange blossom water and blend to a paste.*

2 *Smooth the mask over your face, avoiding the areas round the eyes and mouth. Leave for about 15 minutes until almost dry.*

3 *Rub your fingers over your face to flake the mask away, then rinse with warm water. Splash with cold water, then pat dry. Store any leftover mixture in the fridge and use within a week.*

CREAMY FENNEL MASK FOR DRY SKIN

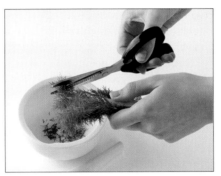

1 *Snip the leafy fronds from a head of fennel and cut into small pieces. Place in a pestle and mortar and bruise the fronds slightly to release the juices.*

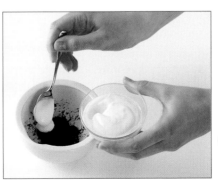

2 *Add 4 tsp of fresh soured cream to the bruised fennel leaves and mix together until evenly blended.*

3 *Smooth the mask gently over your face, avoiding the areas round the mouth and eyes. Leave on for about 15 minutes. Rinse your face thoroughly with warm water and pat dry with a soft towel. Finish by applying a soothing herbal moisturiser to the face and neck.*

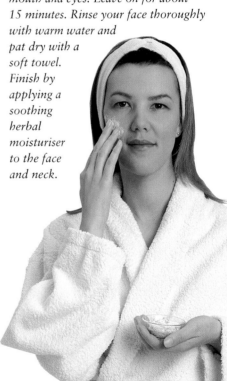

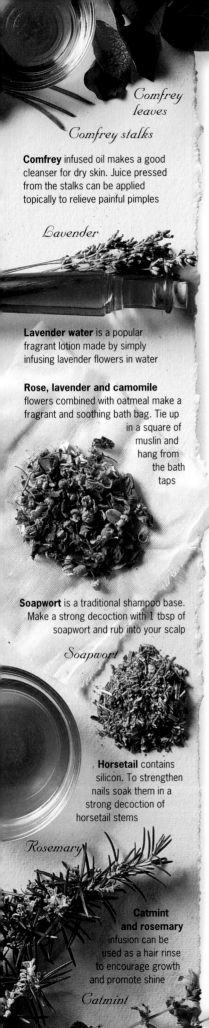

Comfrey infused oil makes a good cleanser for dry skin. Juice pressed from the stalks can be applied topically to relieve painful pimples

Lavender water is a popular fragrant lotion made by simply infusing lavender flowers in water

Rose, lavender and camomile flowers combined with oatmeal make a fragrant and soothing bath bag. Tie up in a square of muslin and hang from the bath taps

Soapwort is a traditional shampoo base. Make a strong decoction with 1 tbsp of soapwort and rub into your scalp

Horsetail contains silicon. To strengthen nails soak them in a strong decoction of horsetail stems

Catmint and rosemary infusion can be used as a hair rinse to encourage growth and promote shine

Herbal Cosmetics

It is easy to make effective herbal cosmetics at home, at a fraction of the price of shop-bought products. Because homemade cosmetics are preservative-free, many of them should be mixed up from fresh herbs immediately before use and are not intended to be stored.

The beneficial effect of oil of evening primrose (*Oenothera biennis*) acts as a catalyst for a group of hormone-like substances, known as prostaglandins, which the body manufactures to combat inflammatory change. This is why a cream containing evening primrose oil is thought to help to relieve eczema and irritated skin in general.

The bark of witch hazel (*Hamamelis mollis* or *virginiana*) produces a powerful astringent which is beneficial for treating bruises. Highly diluted witch hazel is often used as the main ingredient in eye lotions. A little goes a long way, however; too much can stain and damage dry, delicate skin.

Essential oil of rosemary (*Rosmarinus officinalis*) improves the circulation to the skin, which is why fresh rosemary is used as an embrocation or liniment for stiff, aching limbs. This oil is particularly useful for cleansing oily skins. Similarly, lemon balm (*Melissa officinalis*) has good skin penetration and is added to high-quality cosmetic treatments for oily or acne-prone skin.

The petals of many flowers are used as healing agents. Those of the cornflower (*Centaurea cyanus*) are used in gentle toners for dry and sensitive skins, while the petals of the field poppy (*Papaver rhoeas*) have a soothing effect which can reduce itchiness and the discomfort of many skin disorders. Marigold petals (*Calendula officinalis*) contain oils, healing substances and active ingredients which cleanse and decongest the skin, protecting against infection.

Extracts from the root and leaf of burdock (*Arctium lappa*) are known to inhibit the growth of bacteria which commonly inhabit the skin. These extracts can be helpful for oily skin and acne, as can both wild and cultivated thyme. These are strongly antiseptic and so help to preserve a skin preparation as well as protecting the skin from infection or yeast growth. Another therapeutic herb, the horse chestnut or conker tree (*Aesculus hippocastanum*), has astringent and tonic properties, especially to veins and capillaries, and improves circulation, so it is used mainly in strong toners and face masks. In addition, the mildly sedative flowers of this tree may be added to bath water to aid relaxation, while external compresses, lotions and baths of seeds or bark may be applied to varicose veins, to acne and broken blood vessels in the face, and to treat blackheads.

Menthol is a powerful constituent of the essential oils of most species of mint. Very small quantities may be added to specialised skin preparations to cool the skin.

Shampoos and conditioners

A shampoo is a detergent which removes grease, dirt and skin debris from the hair and scalp without harming the skin or hair shaft. A suitable product will improve the appearance of hair and its manageability.

Conditioners improve the 'body' and controllability of hair by emulsifying the surface layer and coating it with long-chain polymers – lengths of joined molecules – and proteins.

A number of plants and their oils have traditionally been associated with a healthy scalp. Rosemary and lavender are well known; many modern 'botanical' shampoos contain more exotic essential oils, such as ylang-ylang, jojoba and vetivert. Nettle has traditionally been used as a hair rinse, and many 'herbal' shampoos include chlorophyll from nettles for its pleasant smell.

Bath oils

Aromatic essences dissolve well in fixed oils derived from plants, but these cannot be used as bath oils because they make the skin very oily and form a greasy film on the bath.

One solution is to blend relatively large quantities of aromatic oils and emulsifiers with a small quantity of fixed oil. The label on the bottle should then indicate that only small amounts should be added to bath water, thus providing good dispersion.

The addition of surfactants will also help. These are surface active agents which are crucial ingredients in the production of any emulsion. They work by reducing the surface tension between substances which normally would not blend, or stay mixed for long. The addition of surfactants results in a homogenous product which mixes throughout the bath water.

THE FUTURE OF PLANTS AS MEDICINE

In the study and practice of herbal medicines, it is crucial not only to understand the constituents and actions of known herbs but also to continue the search for new plants and applications.

While herbal medicines have been used since earliest human existence, it is only in the last 200 years that the development of chemistry has permitted scientists to produce standardised extracts from plants and isolate the 'active' constituents. This process allows greater precision in dosages, and eliminates undesirable characteristics such as an unpleasant taste. Modern herbalism even has its own scientific discipline of pharmacognosy (see page 28), yet estimates of the amount of medicines currently in use that are derived from plants suggest a drop in the last 20 years, probably due to the increased use of synthetic drugs. This does not mean, however, that herbal medicine is in decline.

Research into phytomedicines, as plant remedies are being called, has been accelerating in the last few years. New research and testing has confirmed some established herbal remedies and identified potential new therapeutic uses for others.

Some herbs in particular have been extensively researched; garlic, one of the most researched herbs, has been the subject of nearly 2500 studies. These have built an impressive picture of its medicinal properties.

THE ROLE OF MODERN DRUG COMPANIES
Following early successes in isolating active compounds in plants, the pharmaceutical industry added a number of highly important plant-based drugs to modern medicine. There then followed a period of years when drug companies seemed forced by economic reasons to focus their attention on synthetic, or semi-synthetic compounds that could be easily tested and cheaply produced. In 1980 none of the top 250 pharmaceutical companies had research programmes that

involved plants. Over the last 15 years, however, this picture has changed dramatically as companies became interested once again in looking at plant-derived medicinal products. Today over half of the major drug companies are running research programmes. So far, this revival of interest has not been matched by research support from funding bodies – with the exception of the National Cancer Institute in the USA, which since 1960 has screened at least 35 000 plants at a preliminary level for anti-tumour activity, with some success.

THE CANCER CURE WAITING TO BE DISCOVERED
In the last 40 years only three completely new compounds discovered for use in the treatment of cancer have been approved in the West as official drugs. Two of these, the chemicals vincristine and vinblastine, came from the same plant: the Madagascan periwinkle (*Catharanthus roseus*). The third compound, taxol, was isolated from a species of Pacific yew (*Taxus brevifolia*) and researchers had to wait nearly 20 years before it was approved by the Food and Drug Administration (FDA) in America.

NEW HOPE
More plant extracts are coming to light as remedies for disease. The Australian Moreton Bay chestnut *is currently being researched as a cure for AIDS.*

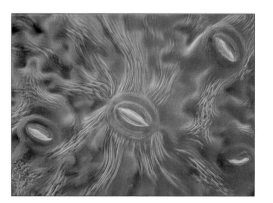

CELLULAR RESEARCH
Electron micrographs, such as this one of an elder leaf, help biologists to study the cellular composition of herbs in order to isolate active ingredients for use in modern medicine.

43

PRESERVING THE ENVIRONMENT

Given the biological diversity of rain-forest ecosystems throughout the world, and their potential to provide important medicines, the rate at which rain forests are being destroyed has caused increasing alarm in recent years. Pressure to expand agriculture is largely responsible for the destruction of areas of the Amazon. Farmers set fire to sections of the forest then fell the remaining trees and undergrowth with earth-moving equipment. Once clear the land is given over to pasture, but conservationists warn that such destruction threatens the forest as a whole through soil degradation and erosion, and the previous biological diversity may never be regenerated.

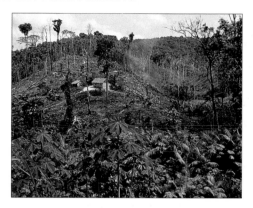

ENDANGERING THE FUTURE?
The rain-forest ecosystem is surprisingly fragile and the plant, insect and animal populations that have survived in harmony for millennia are currently under threat from agricultural expansion.

THE MODERN SHAMAN

One of the most unusual areas of research in recent years has been the development of ethnobotanical studies – the study of traditional uses of plants and their importance to society.

In the rain forests of Central and South America, local healers often use a mixture of local herbal remedies to cure their patients. Their knowledge of local flora is enormous and can lead to surprising breakthroughs in modern scientific research. Indeed, some shamanic herbal remedies are being researched as potential remedies for major modern diseases such as cancer and AIDS.

Out of the 35 000 plants screened for anti-tumour activity this may not appear to be a very high success rate. When researching cancer-fighting compounds it is important that the efficacy of a new compound is clearly established, that it meets stringent safety requirements and that its benefits are proven. Add to this the length of time taken to reach approved-drug status, which can include years of testing, and the thousands of synthetic compounds that are also tested, and the figures fall into perspective.

EXPLORING THE RAIN FORESTS

The extensive rain forests of South and Central America are among the most biodiverse environments on Earth, and possess immense medicinal potential. The South American rain forests offer the richest variety of tropical vegetation found anywhere in the world. So far 25 000 plant species have been identified, but estimates of the number in existence reach to over a million. About one-third of the rain forest flora consists of epiphytes – plants which grow high up on the trunks and branches of the trees. As each tree may have its own unique epiphyte species, the variety is enormous.

Some of our most powerful modern drugs, such as quinine from cinchona, have already come from the few South American plant species investigated so far. Current official plant-derived drugs are obtained from less than one hundred plant species.

GENETIC ENGINEERING

In the last few years, a whole new area of science has come into being – genetics. Scientists can now identify genes in both animals and plants which are relevant to growth, health and well-being.

In the current study of genetics, a great deal of time is being directed at identifying human genes, relating genes to specific disorders, and cloning genes. The hope is that these discoveries will help to determine treatments for, say, cancerous growths.

The other main branch of genetic research focuses on plant genes. The aim of this area of genetics is to support conservation and further the development of genetically bred food crops in the hope of diminishing food shortages in the future.

Designing new medicinal plants

The great majority of genetic research on plants is focused on agricultural and economic needs. Much of the work involves identifying endangered species and building up gene banks – stores of genetic material – which can be used in the future development of stronger, more plentiful crops. Almost inevitably, the focus is on major economic crops rather than medicinal plants, but our knowledge about the therapeutic effects of foodstuffs themselves has expanded enormously in the 1990s through both genetic and other scientific research. It is now recognised that dietary changes can

Using Herbs for

Natural Pain Relief

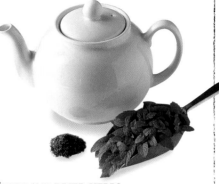

Herbs can be used at home in the form of teas, tablets or compresses for the treatment of many minor aches and pains. If a pain persists or worsens, however, you should always seek qualified medical advice.

The plant world contains some of the most powerful painkillers in existence, such as the opium poppy from which all the opiate drugs are made. There are many herbs that act gently to reduce inflammation, ease tension or soothe pain, which can be used as self-help remedies for many everyday aches. Teas can be made from fresh or dried herbs, generally allowing two heaped dessertspoons of dried or four of fresh herbs to a pint of boiling water.

Effective painkillers
Aspirin, our most commonly used painkiller, was derived from chemicals found naturally in the bark of willow trees. Tablets containing extracts of willow (*Salix alba* or *S. nigra*) may be used to relieve minor pains, while other plants which contain related compounds can also be used, the most common being meadowsweet (aspirin itself was named after an older Latin name for meadowsweet, *Spiraea*). This herb makes a fairly pleasant tea, which can be drunk to ease muscular or joint pains.

Headaches
Relieve recurrent headaches with feverfew (*Tanacetum parthenium*) tablets, taken when necessary. Tension headaches can be eased with a cup of lime blossom (*Tilia europea*) tea to help you to relax;

FRESH AND DRIED HERBS
To make a herbal infusion you will need to use twice as much fresh herb as dried because the dried herb is concentrated.

this can be mixed with peppermint (*Mentha piperita*) to aid digestion if that is also affected.

Indigestion
For indigestion due to inflammation of the digestive system, a cup of warm tea made from the flowers of camomile (*Chamomilla recutita*) can be helpful; for bloating caused by flatulence try peppermint tea. Both these herbs are so popular as self-help remedies that ready-made tea bags are widely available in shops.

MENSTRUAL CRAMPS

Cramping period pains can often be eased by a cup of hot lemon balm (*Melissa officinalis*) tea, which can also settle a painful nervous stomach. A compress over the lower abdomen is another excellent way of using herbs to reduce period pains; the classic herb is cramp bark, or guelder rose (*Viburnum opulus*). Simmer 25 g (1 oz) of the root bark in 600 ml (1 pint) of water for 10 minutes, strain and soak a pad in it. Apply the hot pad to your abdomen. A lavender (*Lavandula vera*) infusion can be used in the same way.

SOOTHING A TOOTHACHE

The pain caused by sensitive teeth or acute toothache can be relieved by topically applying a tincture of myrrh or oil of cloves to the painful area. Although this will offer short term pain relief it is important that any underlying problem, such as a cavity or gum infection, be diagnosed and, where necessary, treated by a dentist as soon as is possible.

SOOTHING CLOVES
At the first twinge of pain from toothache take a clean piece of cotton wool, soak it in oil of cloves and apply it to the affected area. Keep the pad pressed against the area until pain subsides. Pain relief should be almost immediate.

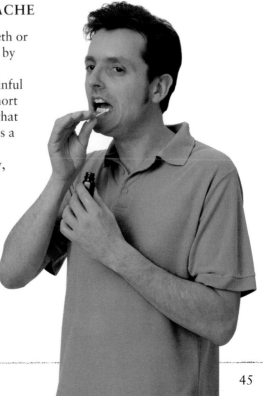

Herbal Myths

Corn has always been a powerful symbol of society's reliance on a successful harvest. In Europe, a common symbol was the pagan corn dolly which was ritualistically sacrificed each year to the gods of the harvest, and later became an accepted figure in the Christian Harvest Festival.

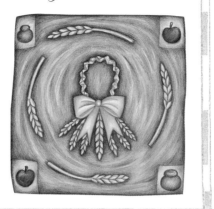

bring about great benefits in protection against disease, including cancers of the stomach, intestines or bowel. For example, several studies have indicated that regular consumption of garlic significantly reduces the incidence of gastro-intestinal cancers (see page 89), and that eating chilli peppers may help to protect against stomach cancers (see page 98).

LOOKING TO THE FUTURE, LEARNING FROM THE PAST

The future of herbal medicine lies in combining the best of traditional skills and experience with the careful exploitation of modern developments in scientific research.

The World Health Organisation (WHO) has been active for several years in promoting the development of traditional medicine. It estimates that 80 per cent of the world's population currently relies on traditional medicine for primary health care and that the great majority of this medicine is derived from plants.

The WHO also considers practitioners of herbal medicine to be an important part of world health care resources and as such it is concerned to improve the standards of safety, effectiveness and quality of herbal treatments. To this end, the WHO is involved in promoting national programmes of analysis, screening, research and education.

The process of screening and testing new treatment applications or new plants now takes place largely in cell lines – using human cells in laboratories for testing the effects of substances, rather than using people or animal testing.

Research into the therapeutic use of plants has become a worldwide venture with more and more of the world's scientists realising the potential of plant remedies.

In the UK and Germany since the late 1970s research has led to developments in the use of traditional remedies such as feverfew (*Tanacetum parthenium*) for the treatment of migraines and St John's wort (*Hypericum perforatum*) for depression.

In China, a great deal of research has gone into the plant *Artemisia annua*, which contains the compound artemisin. This compound is promising to be the newest and most effective antimalarial drug discovered so far. In India, the plant *Coleus forskolin* is being researched for its potential use in the treatment of glaucoma and hypertension.

WILL YOUR DOCTOR PRESCRIBE YOU HERBS?

The somewhat surprising answer is that your doctor already prescribes herbs because many conventional drugs are derived from plants. In many countries, although not so much in the UK, doctors prescribe herbal medicines directly, either as standardised extracts, such as EGb 761 from ginkgo which has been extensively researched for treatment of circulatory disorders, or in their original states or as recognised herbal remedies, such as an infusion of lemon balm (*Melissa officinalis*) to ease premenstrual tension because it works more safely and cheaply than other drugs.

FUTURE MEDICINE

According to geneticists and molecular biologists, the future of drug discovery lies in the scientists' ability to manipulate human genes and develop synthetic drugs custom-made for certain diseases. However, this may be a long way off. It seems foolish, therefore, to ignore the plant kingdom as a potential source of new medicines while we wait for the geneticists to realise the potential of their work. Given the huge numbers of plants in the world there is room for optimism that effective medicines for many modern diseases will be found through such research.

CHAPTER 3

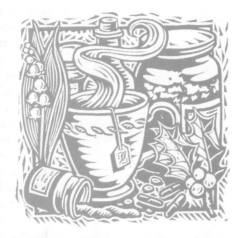

USING HERBS SAFELY

Centuries of using herbs for their medicinal properties have filtered out most that are toxic, leaving only the safe varieties in general use. Herbs like camomile and mint are taken regularly by millions as infusions or condiments, and dangers or side effects are very uncommon. Some herbs, however, are less gentle in their actions, and must therefore be used with caution.

FINDING AND PREPARING HERBS

To use herbs safely and effectively your raw plant material, whether fresh or dried, must be of medicinal quality and not adulterated or replaced by an inferior substitute.

FREEZING
To kill any insect larvae that may be in your herbs – particularly in roots or flower heads – wrap the herb in a polythene bag and place it in the freezer for a few days. The frozen larvae will drop off the herb and be caught in the bag. These can be shaken out and discarded before the herb is used.

The majority of herbs recommended for home use have a gentle action, are considered safe, and are generally only suitable for simple remedies or gentle relief from symptoms. Professional herbalists are able to treat a greater diversity of disorders and have access to a far wider range of herbs, some of which are highly toxic and even lethal if wrongly administered. The better you know your herbs, and your symptoms, the less chance you have of making a mistake.

If you intend to treat yourself with herbal remedies there are a few simple precautions you should take to ensure the best treatment possible. When you first come across a herb, examine it carefully, noting its colour, smell and appearance. Herbs in good condition should retain most of their colour and smell. Compare it, fresh or dried, to a picture of the living plant. At first you may see little resemblance, but soon you will be able to pick out distinctive features like leaf tips, stalks, and even stigmas and stamens. Dried plants should preserve most of the detail of the fresh plant. Avoid herbs that appear dusty. They may be old, or have been exposed to light, air, or infested with insects.

Treating infestation

Normally your supplier will have treated the herbs in some way to counteract infestation by insects. Most imported herbs, other than organically grown ones, are deep frozen, irradiated or treated with ethylene oxide, any of which will decontaminate them.

WHERE TO BUY HERBS

Only buy herbs from a reputable source. Some herbs are hard to grow and wild plants can be scarce or inaccessible. These factors put up costs, making it tempting to substitute or adulterate dried or powdered herbs with a cheaper, similar looking material. Official standards for purity ensure that herbs are not deliberately adulterated, that they contain a good level of active constituents (to prevent the extraction of valuable essential oils before sale, for example) and that they are in a reasonable condition. These standards are rigorously applied in the UK to herbs in licensed herbal medicines.

QUALITY CONTROL OF HERBS

The regulation of dried herbs or herbs in unlicensed medicines (medicines that have not passed necessary pharmaceutical tests or proved their worth) is less stringent than for licensed medicines. This means that adulteration and contamination by bacteria or heavy metals, like lead and cadmium from polluted air, soil or water, is not unknown. Nevertheless, unlicensed medicines are covered by normal trading standards, requiring that material is fit for sale and consumption, and is what it purports to be. Under UK legislation, medicinal claims cannot be made for unlicensed medicines, although descriptions such as 'refreshing' or 'relaxing', or indications as to when best to take a product are acceptable.

Established herbal suppliers and manufacturers in the UK maintain high standards, however. Most belong to the British Herbal Medicines Association, which is involved in setting European standards for herbal labelling and quality. Such suppliers are careful of their reputation, as are the many

THE ANATOMY OF PLANTS

Being aware of the parts of plants used in herbalism and the different treatments that each requires can help you to understand the method needed for a chosen treatment. If one remedy requires angelica root and another saffron stamens, understanding the structure of plants can help you to judge that the saffron remedy will require less preparation than the angelica root because stamens are soft aerial parts while roots are hard and woody.

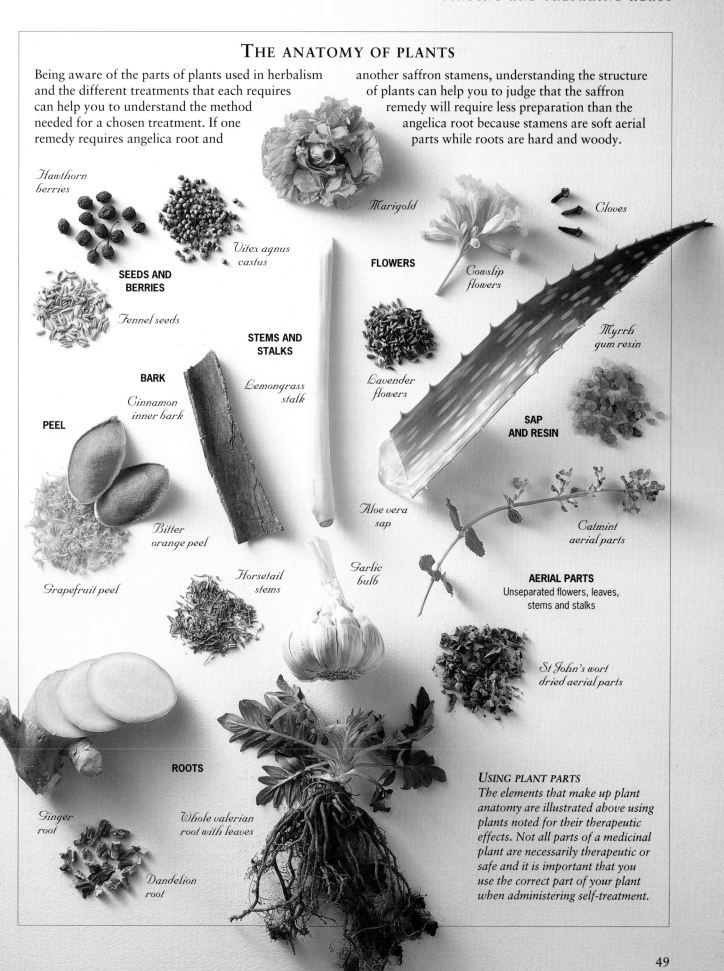

Hawthorn berries

Vitex agnus castus

SEEDS AND BERRIES

Fennel seeds

Marigold

FLOWERS

Cowslip flowers

Cloves

Lavender flowers

STEMS AND STALKS

Lemongrass stalk

Myrrh gum resin

BARK

Cinnamon inner bark

PEEL

Bitter orange peel

Grapefruit peel

SAP AND RESIN

Aloe vera sap

Catmint aerial parts

Horsetail stems

Garlic bulb

AERIAL PARTS
Unseparated flowers, leaves, stems and stalks

St John's wort dried aerial parts

ROOTS

Ginger root

Whole valerian root with leaves

Dandelion root

USING PLANT PARTS
The elements that make up plant anatomy are illustrated above using plants noted for their therapeutic effects. Not all parts of a medicinal plant are necessarily therapeutic or safe and it is important that you use the correct part of your plant when administering self-treatment.

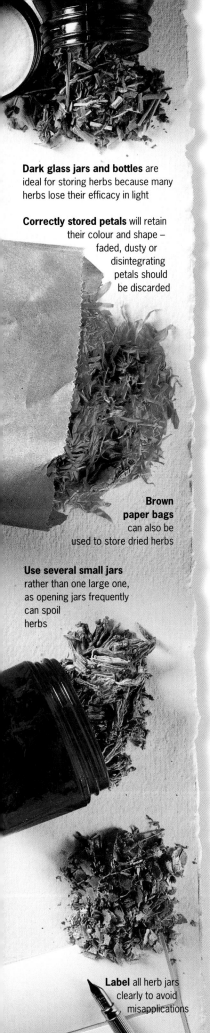

Dark glass jars and bottles are ideal for storing herbs because many herbs lose their efficacy in light

Correctly stored petals will retain their colour and shape – faded, dusty or disintegrating petals should be discarded

Brown paper bags can also be used to store dried herbs

Use several small jars rather than one large one, as opening jars frequently can spoil herbs

Label all herb jars clearly to avoid misapplications

Storing and Labelling

To ensure the best preparations it is important that herbs and herbal products are treated, stored and labelled correctly, both by suppliers and by consumers. If these steps are ignored you may find that remedies and preparations are substandard and may even be dangerous.

shops supplying herbs and herbal medicines. Better shops deal with reputable suppliers only and are knowledgeable about the products they sell and keen to refer customers for professional consultation. Medical herbalists are usually happy to give advice about herbs and herbal products if you want to check the safety or suitability of a remedy.

REGULATIONS IN OTHER COUNTRIES

Herbs are perceived very differently from one country to another. In Germany about 130 herbs are licensed as medicines, with strict standards for composition and purity. A very wide range of teas and other herbal products is available, and the licensing procedure for new products using approved herbs is relatively straightforward. The herbal medicine industry competes seriously with the major drug companies and supplies a high proportion of GP prescriptions.

In the US, herbs are not generally viewed as medicines but as foods, and the trade is often loosely regulated, although this varies from state to state. One result of this arrangement is that quite powerful and sometimes dangerous herbs can go on sale with no labelling or regulation, which is a cause for concern of the Food and Drug Administration. Another is that the potential to develop and market useful herbal products is often wasted because the public is sceptical of herbal remedies. The situation in the UK is somewhere between that in the USA and in Germany. Herbs with a known risk of toxicity are not approved for general sale: except for a few which are available to practitioners, it is an offence to supply unapproved herbs.

A major problem for legislators is that herbs are quite different both from foods (or food additives) and drugs, but are usually put into one of these classifications. In Australia this problem has been addressed by the Traditional Medicines Evaluation Committee, which includes practitioners of

traditional medicine as well as doctors and chemists. Thus, for example, while ginseng is classified as a food for beverage use in the US, and an over-the-counter medicine in Germany and Switzerland, in Australia it is classed as a therapeutic substance and is regulated accordingly.

STORING HERBS TO KEEP THEM FRESH

Herbs must be properly dried before storage, but even so their medicinal properties will eventually fade. Careful storage will keep most herbs in good condition for up to twelve months or so.

Two factors make herbs deteriorate. The first is physical – moisture, heat, air, light and contaminants in the air such as heavy metals like lead can penetrate the herbs. To minimise these effects herbs should be kept dry, cool and dark. Ideally, the temperature should stay below 15°C (60°F).

The second is biological. All sorts of organisms can attack herbs, including bacteria, fungi, insects, rats and mice. In the case of bacteria and fungi, they need moisture to thrive, but the others just need access to the herb. A good solution is to pack the herbs into a secure, airtight container, for example a dark glass jar with a tight-fitting lid. Dry paper in the jar will help to absorb any moisture and keep the herbs fresh.

You should put a date on your container when you fill it, and refill it only when it is empty. Discard – or find another use for – herbs over a year old. As a general rule, the fresher the herb, the better it will work medicinally. However, culinary herbs over a year old can still be used to flavour stews, and herbs like lavender or camomile make a soothing bath. Lavender or hops can be made into a herb pillow to help you to sleep; old hops are actually better than fresh ones for this because the flowers of the female plant, the stroibles, change with age as the constituents oxidise.

HERBAL PREPARATIONS FOR INTERNAL USE

Oral herbal remedies are usually taken in liquid form: infusions, decoctions, tinctures, juices and syrups, and the herbs need to be carefully prepared to avoid destroying their medicinal properties (see pages 75 to 80). Each form has advantages and disadvantages. Tinctures are better than infusions and decoctions for extracting the volatile oils from herbs. Tinctures and syrups also preserve the herb better than dry storage, whereas infusions and decoctions can only be kept fresh in the refrigerator for a couple of days, and juices for a week or so.

The medicinal substances in plants are generally either water or oil soluble. Water-soluble compounds occur in the fluid inside or outside of the plant cell and oil-soluble compounds are often in special glands, in flowers or seeds, or in cell walls and are therefore more difficult to extract. Adding hot water to the herbs for infusions and decoctions extracts mainly water-soluble components of the plant, like glycosides, tannins and flavonoids. The heat does extract some volatile oils, however, and aromatic herbs – like thyme and camomile – should be prepared in a covered container to prevent the oils from evaporating.

Prolonged heat changes the properties of some constituents, so decoctions – made by simmering herbs – should generally be used only for woody material, like tormentil root. Some water-based constituents, like silicates, starch and mucilage, found in horsetail or marshmallow root, can only be extracted by hours of soaking in water.

Retaining essential oils

Some herbs, such as elecampane and lemon balm, lose most of their essential oil even at a moderate heat, and a fresh tincture or a syrup made by cold infusion are excellent ways to preserve their properties.

Another way to prepare herbs that are best used fresh is to extract the juice. Fresh plant juices are now becoming quite widely available in many health food shops, but you can also make your own at home with a juice extractor.

HERBAL PREPARATIONS FOR EXTERNAL USE

For external use, herbs are usually prepared as lotions, which are water based, as infused oils, or as ointments or creams (see page 79). Ointments and creams are made up of tiny droplets of oily liquids that are mixed with and dispersed in a watery medium, so they can incorporate both water-soluble and oil-soluble constituents.

Infused oils generally keep very well but creams need refrigeration and some form of preservative, herbal or otherwise, if they are to last for more than a few weeks. Always discard herbal remedies if they are old or show signs of ageing or mould.

READING THE SIGNS OF FRESHNESS

Before applying a herbal remedy, always check that there are no signs of ageing, discoloration or mould. Depending on the preparation, the life span of your remedy will be limited. If you have any reason to suspect that your remedy is not in good condition, discard and replace it.

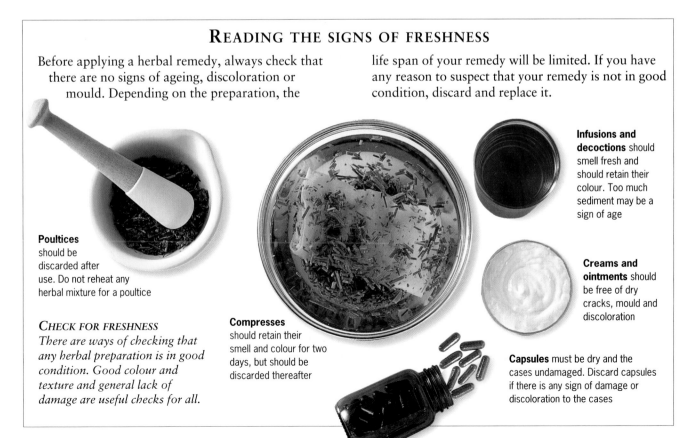

Poultices should be discarded after use. Do not reheat any herbal mixture for a poultice

CHECK FOR FRESHNESS
There are ways of checking that any herbal preparation is in good condition. Good colour and texture and general lack of damage are useful checks for all.

Compresses should retain their smell and colour for two days, but should be discarded thereafter

Infusions and decoctions should smell fresh and should retain their colour. Too much sediment may be a sign of age

Creams and ointments should be free of dry cracks, mould and discoloration

Capsules must be dry and the cases undamaged. Discard capsules if there is any sign of damage or discoloration to the cases

CLASSIFYING HERBS BY USE

When a herb has a therapeutic action, its effect is often described using specific terminology. Understanding these terms can be very useful when describing or choosing herbs.

It is important when choosing a herbal remedy to pick the herbs that are best suited to your symptoms and least likely to cause any problems or side effects. Becoming familiar with the terms used to describe the actions of herbs will help you to understand their effects and help you to choose the best remedy for your condition.

Once you have selected a herb that will relieve your problem, find out the other actions of the herb in question and any cautions and contraindications. It may be that the carminative you plan to use to ease your pregnancy-related indigestion in fact should be avoided by women during pregnancy.

HERBS AND DIGESTIVE PROBLEMS
Possibly the best known and most widely used herbal remedies are those that prevent or relieve digestive disorders.

A herb that stimulates gastric juices and other digestive functions is described as having a bitter action. Bitters are taken to promote digestion and stimulate appetite and can help to relieve acute complaints such as indigestion. Reactions to food allergies will also respond well to bitter herbs as they encourage digestion.

Indigestion and colic can be eased with carminative herbs as these help to relieve and expel flatulence while also calming intestinal spasms and soothing the gut wall. Herbs that generally calm the stomach are called stomachic and may be used to relieve many digestive disorders.

For mild constipation a herbalist would recommend aperient herbs to gently stimulate the normal evacuation of the bowel, although laxatives are also used. Laxatives encourage an abnormal evacuation of the

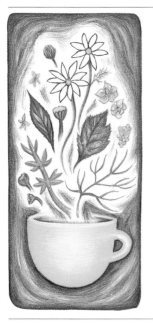

THERAPEUTIC ACTIONS OF HERBS

The chart over the next four pages offers examples of herbs that have particular therapeutic actions, and descriptions of those actions. When you have selected

your herb, carefully follow the instructions for preparation and dosage in Chapters 4, 5 and 6 to achieve the maximum benefit from your remedies.

TERM	ACTION	HERB EXAMPLE
Abortifacient	Increases the risk of or causes abortions or miscarriages	Thuja
Adaptogenic	Improves body's adaptability to cope with stress	Ginseng
Alterative	Speeds up or slows down the body's metabolism as needed	Red clover
Analgesic	Relieves pain	Willow bark
Anodyne	Relieves pain	Cloves
Anthelmintic	Destroys and expels intestinal worms	Wormwood
Anticatarrhal	Combats and relieves congestion in the respiratory tract	Marshmallow
Antiemetic	Suppresses or relieves vomiting and feelings of nausea	Fennel

bowel by irritating the lining of the upper intestine. This causes a reflex action in the digestive tract which stimulates the muscles in the bowel and increases their activity. For a more intensely laxative action to relieve severe constipation a herbalist would recommend a cathartic herb to produce positive bowel evacuation.

Exceptionally laxative herbs that cause a copious movement and evacuation of the bowel are called purgatives. These have a violent effect and should be used with extreme caution.

A cholagogue stimulates the liver to produce bile, which is necessary for healthy digestion. Cholagogue herbs are generally recommended to treat liver disease.

Any substance that suppresses or relieves vomiting or feelings of nausea is called an antiemetic. Care should be taken when using antiemetics; vomiting can be the body's way of clearing unwanted or dangerous substances from the stomach.

An aperitive or exigenic herb can be taken to revive diminished appetite, which may be the result of a minor feverish illness or stress. Normal appetite usually returns of its own accord after the underlying condition has been cured, but a gentle aperitive action may help to bring this about more quickly.

Anthelmintic and vermicidal herbs are used by herbalists to destroy and expel intestinal worms while antiprotozoal herbs kill larger infective parasites such as the protozoa that cause malaria.

DID YOU KNOW?

Dandelion has achieved a widespread notoriety for its diuretic properties. The French call the plant *pissenlit*, and the old English name – piss-a-bed – has equally obvious connotations. At one time it was believed that simply picking the plant would cause you to wet the bed.

HERBS FOR UROGENIC DISORDERS

Urogenital problems such as cystitis or menstrual pain usually respond well to herbal remedies and there are some herbs that are particularly suited to urogenic complaints. Diuretics, for example, provoke an increase in the flow of urine, either by increasing blood flow to the kidneys or by reducing the amount of water reabsorbed by them. Diuretic herbs provide effective relief from urinary infections.

Herbs that increase the risk of or cause miscarriages are called abortifacients. These can damage a foetus but will not completely terminate a pregnancy and should never be taken in an attempt to achieve a termination. A partial or unsuccessful termination can be very dangerous and distressing for both foetus and mother. Some abortifacients may have other properties but should never be taken by pregnant women to treat other disorders. The term emmenagogue is sometimes applied to abortifacients because they can induce menstrual discharge.

TERM	ACTION	HERB EXAMPLE
Anti-infective	Prevents infection	Echinacea
Antiprotozoal	Kills larger infective parasites	Cinchona
Antipyretic	Counteracts and reduces fever	Meadowsweet
Antispasmodic	Relieves the intensity of excessive muscle contractions	Cramp bark
Antitussive	Relieves coughing	Wild cherry bark
Aperient	Mildly laxative – stimulates the normal evacuation of the bowel	Dandelion
Aperitive or exigenic	Revives diminished appetite	Gentian
Astringent	Dries and creates a protective layer on exposed skin and mucous membranes	Tormentil
Bacteriocidal	Attacks and destroys bacteria	Thyme
Bacteriostatic	Inhibits or retards the growth of bacterial infections	Echinacea
Bitter	Stimulates gastric juices and other digestive functions	Wormwood
Carminative	Relieves flatulence, calms intestinal spasms, soothes the gut wall	Fennel

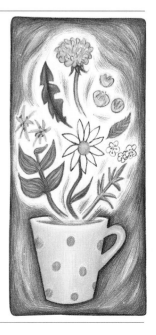

▶ *p. 54*

HERBS AND THE SKIN

Many skin conditions can be effectively treated with herbal remedies. The remedies are usually topically applied in the form of an ointment, cream or poultice.

Herbs with astringent properties create a protective layer on exposed skin and the mucous membranes which protects against irritation and inflammation.

Emollient herbs soothe the skin and can be used to relieve rashes. They tend to have a gentle action and few, if any, cause side effects. Rubefacient herbs cause the skin to redden and become warm as they dilate the blood vessels beneath the skin's surface. The increased blood flow improves the cleansing and nourishing of the tissue.

An alterative herb changes the body's metabolism to increase the efficiency of, among other things, elimination of toxins that can lead to skin disease.

Any herbs that promote wound healing are described as vulnerary. They are generally applied topically to the damaged area.

HERBS AND EMOTIONAL HEALTH

Herbs are commonly used for the therapeutic effect they have on the nervous system, whether to induce relaxation or stimulate positive emotions. An adaptogen, for example, helps to maintain a healthy 'stress response' and improves both mental and physical resistance to stress. Adaptogenic herbs are often recommended for stress-related disorders such as insomnia.

Conditions that may stem from nervous tension, such as irritable bowel syndrome and some migraines, may respond well to a relaxant. These herbs reduce muscular and nervous tension without affecting mental alertness in the way a conventional tranquilliser would. Sedatives act on the nervous system to reduce nervous activity and, unlike relaxants, these may cause drowsiness and dull mental alertness.

Herbs that are described as thymoleptic have an antidepressant action and can help to lift mood.

HERBS AND THE BLOOD

Angina, varicose veins and blood pressure problems can all react well to herbal treatment. Hypertensive herbs, those that raise blood pressure, can be used to relieve poor circulation and blood pressure-related dizziness and fainting, while hypotensive herbs, those that lower blood pressure, can relieve hypertension and related disorders, such as an increased risk of heart disease. Herbs that reduce blood sugar levels are described as hypoglycaemic.

Herbs with a vasodilatory action relax and open blood vessels allowing the blood to flow more freely. These are recommended for conditions such as angina.

Styptic or haemostatic herbs act to stop bleeding and other discharges, such as mucus, both internally and externally. This action is effective whether the herbs are applied topically or taken internally.

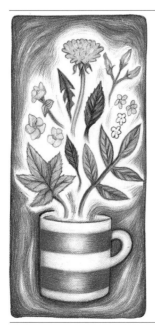

TERM	ACTION	HERB EXAMPLE
Cathartic	Intensely laxative, purges the bowel	Senna
Cholagogue	Stimulates the liver to excrete bile	Goldenseal
Demulcent	Soothes sore or infected membranes	Slippery elm
Diaphoretic	Increases perspiration, helps to reduce a fever	Elder flower
Diuretic	Provokes an increase in the flow of urine	Dandelion leaf
Emmenagogue	Induces menstrual discharge	Mugwort
Emollient	Soothes the skin	Marshmallow
Expectorant	Stimulates bronchial passages, soothes respiratory tract, relieves bronchial spasm, loosens catarrhal secretions	Mullein
Febrifuge	Reduces a fever	Meadowsweet
Fungicidal	Suppresses and kills fungi	Garlic
Galactogogue	Promotes the flow of milk in nursing mothers	Fennel
Hypertensive	Increases blood pressure	Liquorice
Hypoglycaemic	Lowers blood sugar	Garlic

HERBS AND RESPIRATION

Inhalants are an obvious choice for treating respiratory disorders because the active constituents are applied directly to the affected area. Other preparations, however, can also be very effective. Anticatarrhal herbs help to combat and relieve congestion in the respiratory tract. A build-up of phlegm secreted from the mucous membranes can block the passage of air to the lungs and cause difficulties in breathing. Anticatarrhal herbs will help to clear the airways.

Antitussive herbs relieve coughing. Most herbal treatments for coughs kill bacteria and loosen and expel mucus.

Disorders of the bronchial passages, such as asthma or a cough, that are caused by excess phlegm may respond well to expectorant herbs. These either stimulate activity in the bronchial passages, leading to a more productive cough, or soothe the lining of the upper digestive tract which leads to reflex relief of bronchial spasm and loosens catarrhal excretions.

Any herb described as a demulcent will have a soothing action when applied to sore or infected membranes. These are often used to relieve coughs and sore throats.

HERBS AND GENERAL PROBLEMS

Many herbs have wide-reaching actions which can be applied to a diverse number of health complaints in different parts of the body. Herbs that relieve pain without side effects such as loss of consciousness are said to be analgesic or anodyne. These may be applied externally to the affected area or taken internally.

Any herb that acts on a fever and reduces a high temperature is called a febrifuge. Such herbs either induce sweating in the body which dries on the skin and lowers the overall temperature of the patient; or they have a directly cooling effect on the system. Diaphoretic herbs also promote sweating and can reduce a temperature. Conditions that share the symptoms of a fever, such as flu, can be relieved by antipyretic herbs.

A herb described as having a bacteriocidal action attacks and destroys bacteria in the body whereas herbs that inhibit or retard the growth of bacterial infections and prevent bacterial replication are described as bacteriostatic.

Fungicidal herbs act to suppress and kill fungi, such as that which causes athlete's foot, whereas those that act to kill viruses, such as the common cold, are known as viricidal. However, herbs which inhibit and retard the growth of viral infections, by preventing replication as opposed to killing them, are described as virostatic.

A substance that helps to seal body tissues against infection is described as an anti-infective. Herbs with anti-infective actions are often applied topically.

Preventing or curing spasmodic convulsions, spasms or cramps by relieving the intensity of excessive muscle contractions can be achieved with antispasmodic herbs.

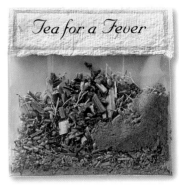

FEBRIFUGAL TEA
A hot infusion made from diaphoretic and febrifugal herbs, such as yarrow, comfrey and cayenne, will increase perspiration and help to reduce a high fever. Place 1 tsp each of dried yarrow and comfrey in a cup, add a pinch of cayenne and pour on hot but not boiling water. Sip one cup four times a day.

TERM	ACTION	HERB EXAMPLE
Hypotensive	Lowers blood pressure	Yarrow
Laxative	Promotes the evacuation of the bowel	Rhubarb
Purgative	Causes a copious movement and evacuation of the bowel	Aloe
Relaxant	Reduces muscular and nervous tension	Cramp bark
Rubefacient	Reddens and warms the skin	Rosemary
Sedative	Reduces nervous activity	Valerian
Stomachic	Comforts the stomach	Comfrey
Styptic or haemostatic	Stops bleeding and other discharge	Agrimony
Thymoleptic	Lifts mood – antidepressant	St John's wort
Vasodilatory	Relaxes and opens blood vessels	Camomile
Vermicidal	Kills intestinal worms	Garlic
Viricidal or virostatic	Kills viruses or retards their growth	Echinacea
Vulnerary	Promotes wound healing	Comfrey

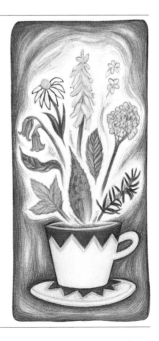

Dangerous herbs

Herbs that are toxic are now well recognised, and herbalism relies on plants with a good safety record and gentle actions. Accidental poisoning, however, is by no means uncommon.

Dangerous or poisonous plants can often be found growing alongside common edible herbs in the countryside, in parks and in gardens, so it is imperative that you are absolutely certain which herb you are gathering.

Some, like foxglove, are very common; some, like yew, have attractive, enticing berries; and others, like fool's-parsley, look very similar to edible plants. For these reasons you must be confident of their identification and properties before using them.

If you have any doubt about plants that you are harvesting or intending to use, avoid them rather than take a risk.

CORRECT IDENTIFICATION
If you decide to harvest your own plants, always look up all the identifying characteristics of any unfamiliar herb in a reliable reference book and then cross-reference it with another book to be absolutely sure. Some edible and poisonous plants can share the same common name, therefore checking against the scientific name is a more reliable indication of what you are picking.

If you are purchasing poisonous herbs from a shop for medicinal use, the herbalist's instructions must be followed exactly. If you experience any adverse reactions, stop taking the herb and seek help immediately from a qualified herbalist or doctor.

The herbs in this section are known to be toxic and should never be used without professional advice.

POISONOUS HERBS
Some poisonous herbs have very powerful emetic or purgative effects, while others can cause paralysis, extreme sedation or heart failure. The majority have been used medicinally in the past in life-threatening circumstances, where modern drugs – the majority of which are toxic in high doses – were unavailable or could not be used. A few of the less toxic plants are still used by medical herbalists, who have the training to use them safely.

COMMON CONFUSIONS
Some dangerous herbs are harder to spot than others and there are a few that are easily confused with common harmless plants, which makes their poisonous nature all the more dangerous.

Daffodil (bulb) *(Narcissus pseudo-narcissus)*
The bulb of a daffodil is similar in shape and size to a small onion but is very toxic. These poisonous bulbs, found in gardens and parks, can cause vomiting and paralysis. Although most plant bulbs look a little like onions, none should be eaten because they can all cause gastric upsets, or worse.

Fool's-parsley *(Aethusa caenapium)*
It is best not to pick any plant in the wild that looks like parsley – many members of the parsley family are poisonous and

PAST LESSONS
Although modern medicine has identified most toxic substances, and found antidotes for many, a number of people suffered in the past due to lack of knowledge about safe doses and toxicity. History is littered with tales of suicides, failed cures and fatal doses of numerous toxic substances, such as the case of Thomas Chatterton (in the painting below by Henry Wallace). The famous English forger-poet poisoned himself with a dose of arsenic.

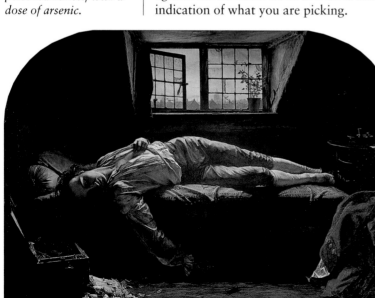

extremely difficult to distinguish from their edible cousins. Although the family includes familiar culinary plants, such as celery, coriander and fennel, it is safest to buy these from reputable suppliers or greengrocers.

All parts of the herb fool's-parsley are poisonous and have a similar deadly action to hemlock. Found on waste and arable land the difference to look for is that common, garden parsley has yellow flowers while fool's-parsley has white ones.

Water dropwort (*Oenanthe aquatica*)
Although generally found in ditches and stagnant water, water dropwort can be mistaken for a parsnip or lovage because its leaves are very similar to both.

All parts are poisonous, especially the fruits, and can cause sweating and irritation or even coma and death.

Water dropwort is probably the most poisonous plant to be found in towns and cities in northern Europe.

POISONOUS HERBS TO AVOID

Most of the dangerous herbs mentioned in the chart below have very obvious toxic effects but are rarely found in the wild. Nevertheless, if you have small children or are planning a family, you should pay particular attention to the plants in your garden or locally that you consider to be simply decorative.

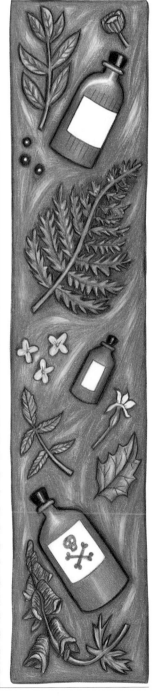

LATIN NAME	COMMON NAMES	POISONOUS PART	EFFECTS	HABITAT
Aconitum napellus	Monkshood, Aconite, Wolfsbane	All parts	Extreme sedation, coma, death	Woods, scrubland, gardens, mountain pastures
Arum maculatum	Lords and ladies	All parts, esp. berries	Severe diarrhoea	Woods, hedgerows
Atropa belladonna	Deadly nightshade	All parts	Delirium, death	Woods, gardens
Chelidonium maius	Greater celandine	All parts	Nausea, dysentery	Hedges, wasteland
Cicuta virosa	Water hemlock, Cowbane	All parts, especially root	Convulsions, death	Ditches, marshes
Daphne mezereum	Mezereon, Flowering spurge	All parts	Severe contact irritation	Woods, gardens
Datura stramonium	Thornapple, Jimson weed	All parts	Toxic and hallucinogenic	Waste land, cultivated ground, gardens
Dryopteris filix-mas	Male fern	All parts	Poisoning, coma, blindness	Forests, shady banks
Helleborus niger	Black hellebore	All parts, especially root	Diarrhoea, vomiting, heart failure	Woods, scrubland, parks, gardens
Helleborus viridis	Green hellebore	All parts, especially root	Diarrhoea, vomiting, heart failure	Woods, scrubland, parks, gardens
Polygonatum odoratum	Solomon's seal	Berries	Nausea, vomiting	Woods, gardens
Prunus laurocerasus	Cherry laurel	Leaves	Paralysis, respiratory failure	Parks, gardens
Sedum acre	Wall-pepper, Biting stonecrop	All parts	Severe irritation	Walls, rocky soils
Senecio jacobaca	Ragwort	All parts	Liver disease	Grassland, gardens
Senecio vulgaris	Groundsel	All parts	Liver disease	Grassland, gardens
Tamus communis	Black bryony	All parts	Gastric irritation, vomiting	Hedges, scrubland
Tanacetum vulgare	Tansy	All parts	Gastric irritation	Wasteland, hedges

COMMON DANGEROUS HERBS

Many highly dangerous herbs can be found in fields, wooded areas and gardens, by the sides of roads and rivers, and in parks and waste ground. Some have pretty flowers and attractive berries, others bear remarkable resemblances to favourite common garden flowers, but almost all, if taken internally, can cause violent reactions and lead to symptoms ranging from vomiting to delirium, palpitations, hallucinations and even death.

When applied professionally, however, the active properties of these poisonous plants can be used to treat many disorders, from respiratory problems to muscular pain, and should not be dismissed from the domain of herbal medicine. It is never recommended, however, that any of the herbs in this section are harvested or used for self-treatment in any form.

In most instances all parts of the plants are highly poisonous – with some parts having a more violent action than others – and should be used only with strict professional medical supervision. In the event of accidental poisoning it is important that the patient receives immediate medical attention and that, where possible, the doctor is told which plant is involved.

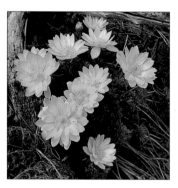

Yellow pheasant's eye

Adonis vernalis YELLOW PHEASANT'S EYE

Also known as false hellebore, this green-ribbed plant grows in gardens and cornfields and produces single, bright yellow flowers in the spring.

Although all parts of this herb are extremely toxic, it has become favoured in professional use as a heart sedative and a treatment for hypertension. It has also been found to contain certain active ingredients similar to those found in foxglove which can help to increase the efficiency of the heart. Nevertheless, no type of pheasant's eye should ever be gathered for home use or administered as self-treatment.

Poisoning from the plant can lead to diarrhoea, vomiting, paralysis and heart failure. Yellow pheasant's eye is rare and is legally protected in many parts of western Europe.

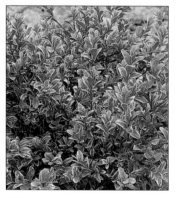

Box

Buxus sempervirens BOX

A small evergreen tree or shrub, box produces yellow-green flowers in spring, has tough, toxic wood and oblong, glossy, dark green leaves. Although rarely found in the wild in the UK, box can often be found in parks and gardens, nurtured as an ornamental plant. All parts of box are poisonous, but the leaves and seeds are particularly toxic. Box wood has sedative and narcotic properties, but the leaves are very dangerous and have been known to cause death in animals that have eaten them. Homeopaths use a tincture made from fresh box leaves to relieve fevers, urinary tract infections and rheumatism, but the minute quantities used are harmless. Poisoning from box can lead to severe abdominal pain, vomiting and diarrhoea, often with blood. For herbal treatments, box should only be used under professional instruction.

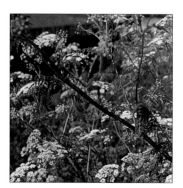

Hemlock

Conium maculatum HEMLOCK

Commonly found in open woods, by roadsides and often near water, hemlock has an off-putting smell that has been likened to mouse urine. This smell and the purple patches that appear on the stem distinguish hemlock from other members of its family (umbellifer), such as parsley. In summer the plant produces clusters of tiny white flowers that form a flat or slightly curved surface or umbel which is distinctive of the umbellifer family and will help with identification. The fruit of hemlock is the most medicinally active part of the plant, but is only used in minute homeopathic doses to relieve pain. In all other cases hemlock is deadly poisonous, especially its green, almost ripe seeds, and should never be harvested or used for any form of self-treatment.

Convallaria majalis LILY OF THE VALLEY

A hardy perennial, lily of the valley grows in any soil, but thrives in humus-rich moist soil such as that found in woodland and valleys. It has white flowers that are drooping and bell-shaped and have a sweet smell which makes it a popular garden plant. In autumn the lily produces bright red spherical berries which are highly toxic and can cause paralysis and respiratory failure. Children should be particularly warned against handling or eating these attractive berries.

All parts of the lily are extremely poisonous and should never be used for self-medication, although some parts are used by herbalists for their beneficial action on the heart – the lily encourages a slow, regular heartbeat, similar to the action of foxglove.

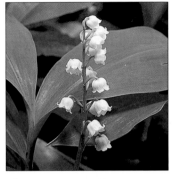

Lily of the valley

Digitalis purpurea FOXGLOVE

This hardy biennial, also considered a short-lived perennial, produces pink, mauve, red or white trumpet-shaped flowers with spotted interiors. Found on heathland and in gardens, all parts of the foxglove are highly toxic when taken internally, yet from this plant comes one of the most widely used and universally recognised heart drugs, digitoxin. Paradoxically, one of the symptoms of digitalis poisoning is an irregular heart action. Other symptoms may include abdominal pain, stomach irritation, nausea, tremors and even death.

Although the deep green oval leaves are sometimes prescribed as treatment for epilepsy and tumours, because of the danger of poisoning it is illegal to give foxglove as an internal preparation unless you are a qualified doctor.

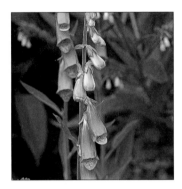

Foxglove

Hyoscyamus niger HENBANE

A woody-stemmed herb found mainly in wasteland and sandy soil, henbane is extremely poisonous and foul smelling. All parts of the herb are covered in a fine down and the flowers are pale yellow and pitcher-shaped with purple veins. Henbane has a violent action that can result in palpitations, respiratory failure, delirium, hallucinations and death. Used by professional herbalists, henbane can be useful in the treatment of digestive, urinary tract and asthmatic spasms. The sticky, grey-green leaves also have pain-relieving properties which can reduce muscular spasms and induce a deep, healing sleep.

Henbane has been widely used in herbalism, homeopathy and also in conventional medicine where the toxic dosage is carefully monitored. The essential oil is sometimes used in creams and liniments for relieving rheumatism.

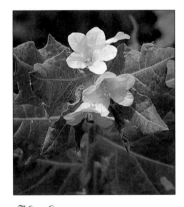

Henbane

Ilex aquifolium HOLLY

Found mostly in parks, gardens and woodland, holly is a popular Christmas plant, because of its bright red winter berries and shiny, rich green leaves. The berries of the holly are toxic, however, and can cause serious bouts of vomiting and diarrhoea. This can be particularly dangerous for children who may find the berries appetising. In professional use, the leaves are infused to help to treat colds and coughs and have diuretic properties that relieve urinary infections. They are also used as a fever remedy and have some therapeutic action in the treatment of jaundice and rheumatism.

Despite its many applications, holly should only be used medicinally under strict professional supervision and should never be used as a self-help treatment or for children.

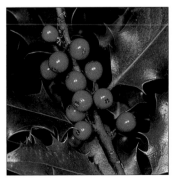

Holly

Laburnum anagyroides LABURNUM

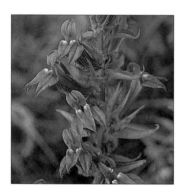

Laburnum

A small deciduous tree, laburnum can be found on mountainsides and in gardens and parks. It produces small yellow flowers in long, drooping groups – giving it its common name, Golden Chain – and in autumn, brown seed pods that cluster along the stems. All parts of the tree are poisonous, particularly the seed pods, so it is important that children are warned not to eat them. Symptoms of poisoning with laburnum include stomach cramps, vomiting, dilated pupils, respiratory failure, dizziness, convulsions and death. An extract of laburnum is sometimes used in conventional medicine to treat hypotension and in homeopathic medicine a preparation of the leaves and flowers is used to relieve neurological and digestive disorders. Laburnum should never be used for self-treatment.

Lobelia inflata LOBELIA

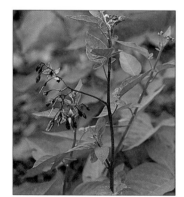

Lobelia

Also known as Indian tobacco, this plant contains certain extracts that are added to antismoking mixtures. These extracts act as a nicotine substitute.

A popular house and garden plant in western Europe, *Lobelia inflata* produces small, pretty, spiky lavender-blue flowers between June and October and has finely serrated, long, narrow leaves. It is the leaves which are poisonous.

More toxic than other members of the lobelia family (campanulaceae), Indian tobacco has an emetic and expectorant action but can cause unpleasant side effects including depression, sweating, nausea and vomiting if taken without strict professional supervision. With proper guidance, however, lobelia can help to relieve a number of disorders, from asthma to backache.

Solanum dulcamara BITTERSWEET

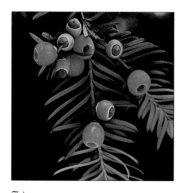

Bittersweet

A shrubby climber, bittersweet, or woody nightshade as it is commonly called, has a slender stem and poisonous berries which are red when ripe.

Most commonly found in woodland, hedgerows and on shingle beaches, its purple flowers have yellow anthers, which can look very pretty in spring.

Unfortunately, although attractive, the plant is highly toxic. The twigs of bittersweet – which taste first bitter and then sweet, hence its name – can cause permanent paralysis of the tongue and loss of speech if ingested.

Used professionally, the plant is widely prescribed by herbalists and homeopaths as a liver tonic and an asthma treatment and can be applied topically to relieve skin disorders. The toxic bittersweet stems also have both diuretic and antirheumatic properties but should never be used as a home remedy.

Taxus baccata YEW

Yew

A slow-growing conifer with a conical shape and domed crown, yew is found in churchyards, ornamental gardens and parks. The leaves are flattened, needle-like and dark green. In autumn, the ripe fruit consists of a seed partially enclosed in a fleshy, bright red 'cup'. Strangely, the red cup is the only part of the yew which is not poisonous, but the seeds and leaves are very toxic. Mild yew poisoning can cause gastroenteritis and collapse, while larger doses can result in sudden death. A tincture of fresh yew leaves is used in homeopathy to treat arthritis, gout, rheumatism, urinary tract infections, heart and liver conditions, but is widely considered too toxic for herbal use, even among professionals. Yew should never be self-administered or used without professional guidance.

MISAPPLICATION AND OVERDOSING

The most common problems in herbal treatment are not side effects – these are rare with herbs that are recommended and approved for general sale – but misapplication.

Self-diagnosis is always potentially dangerous, and herbal medicine can be subtle. Two apparently similar complaints may require different remedies, and the wrong herb may exacerbate a problem.

A few people have allergies to certain herbs, often to a group of herbs that are related botanically, which can cause skin rashes or headaches. If you have a history of allergies, start carefully when taking herbs. Take a low dose of one herb by itself for a few days, rather than taking a mixture. If you are planning to use a herb externally, it is a good idea to carry out a patch test first:

try the remedy out for a day or two on an area of skin that is not inflamed or irritated to see whether that herb gives you any adverse reactions.

If you do get a reaction, stop taking the herb. If the reaction is immediate and external, such as a rash, wash the area thoroughly with clean, warm water and pat dry. If other reactions occur, such as vomiting or chest pains, seek immediate medical advice.

Never try to relieve extreme allergic reactions with other untested herbs; you may exacerbate the symptoms. If you suffer a reaction, seek professional advice.

MAINTAINING SAFE LEVELS

The following remedies are safe as long as the dosage, duration of use and rest periods are adhered to. The rest periods will ensure that there is not a dangerous build-up of the active constituents in your system. It is recommended that you take professional advice before embarking on a course of treatment.

NAME	MAXIMUM DAILY DOSE	DURATION (WEEKS)	REST PERIOD (WEEKS)	CONTRAINDICATIONS/CAUTIONS
Bearberry (*Arctostaphylos uva-ursi*)	3 g	2	2	May cause kidney disease if taken for a long time
Blood root (*Sanguinaria canadensis*)	0.5 g	2	1	Follow professional advice. Avoid during pregnancy/lactation
Broom (*Cytisus spp.*)	3 g	2	1	Follow professional advice
Cascara sagrada (*Cascara sagrada*)	3 g	1	2	Use for a few days at a time before bed
Comfrey (*Symphytum officinalis*)	3 g	4	4	Leaves only for internal use
Ginseng (*Panax spp.*)	2 g	12	4	May cause menstrual problems, nervous tension, heart disease. Avoid with caffeine
Liquorice (*Glycyrrhiza glabra*)	4 g	2	1	May cause hypertension
Lignum vitae (*Guaiacum officinalis*)	2 g	4	2	May cause acute inflammation or allergy
Pokeroot (*Phytolacca americana*)	0.3 g	2	2	Follow professional advice. Avoid during pregnancy
Senna (*Cassia spp.*)	2 g	1	3	Not for colicky constipation. Avoid during pregnancy
Tansy (*Tanacetum vulgare*)	1 g	2	2	Follow professional advice. Avoid during pregnancy

OVERDOSING

Overdoses of toxic herbs are obviously dangerous, but even some milder herbs can have a cumulative ill effect and are best taken only for short periods. Others that are quite safe over long periods in therapeutic dosages can still cause unpleasant sensations or medical complications if taken in too large a dose. Always check if your chosen herbal remedy has a maximum safe dosage or is known to have any contraindications. Also, bear in mind that some herbs may be perfectly safe for most people but are contraindicated for specific conditions such as during pregnancy or for hypertension. If in doubt, always seek professional advice.

The best way to choose the right herb is to find one that is commonly recommended for your condition and then to read as much as you can about it. Pay particular attention to your whole symptom range and the range of actions of the herb and always take the recommended dose for the recommended period of time.

DAILY DOSES

The chart below lists a number of commonly available herbs which require particular care. Although all are on general sale and safe when properly used, you must pay close attention to the dosage. Never exceed the daily dose. Stop treatment and consult your herbalist if you suffer any negative effects.

NAME	MAXIMUM DAILY DOSE	CONTRAINDICATIONS/CAUTIONS
Barberry (Berberis spp.)	2 g	Avoid during pregnancy
Black cohosh (Cimicifuga racemosa)	1 g	Follow professional advice. Avoid during pregnancy
Blue cohosh (Caulophyllum thalictroides)	1 g	Avoid during pregnancy (until labour)
Blue flag (Iris versicolor)	2 g	Discontinue in cases of digestive irritation
Cayenne (Capsicum spp.)	120 mg	Avoid with gastric hyperacidity/acid indigestion
Celery seed (Apium graveolens)	3 g	Avoid during pregnancy
Feverfew (Tanacetum parthenium)	1 g	Avoid during pregnancy
Figwort (Scrophularia spp.)	5 g	Avoid with tachycardia (rapid heartbeat)
Goldenseal (Hydrastis canadensis)	2 g	Avoid during pregnancy. Not for children
Hops (Humulus lupulus)	1 g	Avoid during depressive illness
Juniper (Juniperus spp.)	2 g	Avoid during pregnancy or with kidney disease
Maté (Ilex paraguariensis)	4 g	Stimulating – treat like strong coffee
Mugwort (Artemisia vulgaris)	2 g	Avoid during pregnancy
Oats (Avena sativa)	4 g	Avoid if gluten sensitive
Pasqueflower (Pulsatilla spp.)	0.3 g	Must not be used fresh
Pennyroyal (Mentha pulegium)	3 g	Avoid during pregnancy
Queen's delight (Stillingia sylvatica)	2 g	Not to be used after 2 years storage
Rue (Ruta graveolens)	1 g	Avoid during pregnancy. Irritant and emetic
Sage (Salvia spp.)	3 g	Avoid during pregnancy
Sassafras (Sassafras albidum)	3 g	Do not use oil of sassafras internally
Sweet flag (Acorus calamus)	2 g	Keep within stated dose; avoid isolated oil
Thuja (Thuja occidentalis)	3 g	Avoid during pregnancy
Wild lettuce (Lactuca spp.)	3 g	High doses can be dangerous
Wormwood (Artemisia spp.)	2 g	Avoid during pregnancy

TREATMENT AND SELF-DIAGNOSIS

Herbal treatment often complements conventional medical treatment, but can also interfere with it. You should always inform your doctor or therapist of any medicines you are taking.

Most of our commonest health problems, such as tension headaches, occasional insomnia or colds are minor and familiar and few people consider professional treatment to be necessary. Other disorders, such as hay fever, are seen more as a nuisance than a serious health problem, yet for all these conditions there is effective herbal treatment.

For symptoms that seem serious or that need urgent attention (see page 66) you should see your GP or go to your nearest Accident and Emergency department. They have access to many different resources within the health service, and can refer you directly for tests or to a specialist.

Less urgent conditions can be treated with a visit to a properly trained herbalist. If your problem needs further investigation the herbalist will ask you to consult your GP, and may contact the GP or write a letter for you to take along.

IS IT SAFE TO TAKE HERBS WITH PRESCRIBED DRUGS?

If a condition is serious enough to require professional treatment, you should not add to or modify the treatment without professional supervision. In general, a medical herbalist will know more about interactions between herbs and drugs than a doctor, because few doctors in the UK are familiar with medicinal herbs.

Herbs can often provide a good substitute for your prescription. If your medication is for a minor, self-limiting condition like a cold or hay fever, you can try using herbs. A medical herbalist will tell you whether you can safely replace your doctor's prescription with the herbal treatment, but you should keep your GP informed.

If you are seeing a herbalist as well as taking medicines prescribed by your doctor, the herbalist should advise you about the compatibility of the herbs and medicines, and your herbal prescription should take account of any prescribed drugs. You should take any prescription medicines to the consultation. You should also inform the doctor if you are seeing a herbalist – it is not just courteous but also sensible to keep everyone involved in your treatment aware of each other. Any good complementary practitioner will encourage you to inform other practitioners, or will do so themselves.

CHOOSING A PRACTITIONER

A good practitioner, whether they be a GP, herbalist or other therapist, is always keen to learn more about their branch of medicine and will be genuinely concerned about you and about your condition. He or she should be willing to discuss all aspects of your treatment with you, giving you a clear description of the causes of your condition, what is likely to happen and why. If you get a strong impression that your practitioner has hardly listened to a word you have said, or has dismissed your worries, you should think seriously about looking for someone else.

Reactions to both herbs and drugs always carry a certain amount of unpredictability. You may get side effects to one medicine or another, and new aspects of your condition

---

Mint and Lemongrass Tea
to soothe indigestion

2 tbsp dried peppermint
1 tbsp dried, chopped lemongrass stalk
1 tbsp crushed fennel seeds
1 tbsp dried camomile flowers

■ Place all the herbs together in an airtight tin and shake to mix them thoroughly.
■ To make up the tea, put 1 tsp of the mix in a cup and pour on hot but not boiling water. Leave to infuse for 5 minutes.
■ Take 1 cup after rich, heavy meals to soothe indigestion.

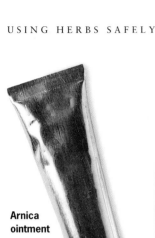

Arnica ointment

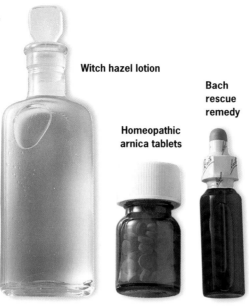

Witch hazel lotion

Homeopathic arnica tablets

Bach rescue remedy

HOLISTIC FIRST-AID
Although there are many situations in which herbal or homeopathic remedies are not recommended, a simple first-aid kit offers immediate relief before medical help arrives. For shock, Bach flower rescue remedy or homeopathic arnica tablets can help. For minor burns and sunburn, distilled witch hazel or aloe vera will relieve pain. Bruises and sprains can be eased with arnica ointment – but apply only to unbroken skin. Lavender oil can help with pain relief.

may come to light. Your treatment may therefore change significantly over time.

However, if you have serious side effects with a particular medicine, or suffer a series of different reactions or unexplained changes in treatment, you should consider a change of practitioner.

A practitioner or GP who suits one patient may, for reasons of personality or professional strengths and weaknesses, not suit another. You need to be able to trust your practitioner both as a person and as a therapist, not only because you are handing her or him responsibility for your health, but also because without that trust you will be less receptive and your treatment will be less

HERBAL REMEDIES *vs.* 'OVER-THE-COUNTER' CURES

Many over-the-counter medicines are highly sugared with little or no real medicinal value, especially syrups and pastilles sold to remedy coughs and sore throats.

This is not to say that many such medicines will not relieve immediate symptoms of minor illnesses, but that many homemade herbal remedies can be used to treat the same conditions and will have a more beneficial overall medicinal effect.

For conditions where medical help is needed, herbal first aid will give just as effective, or ineffective, immediate relief as most conventional over-the-counter first-aid treatments.

effective. One reason for this is that if you don't trust your therapist you may want to stop treatment too early to derive benefit.

SELF-DIAGNOSIS

Going to your GP with a common complaint, such as a cold or diarrhoea, is usually unnecessary as these symptoms tend to disappear after a few days even if left untreated. In instances such as these, self-diagnosis is often perfectly adequate and the use of herbs to alleviate any pain and hasten the healing process is fine.

Problems arise when simple symptoms last for more than a few days or become increasingly worse, when they may be a sign of a more serious underlying illness.

Skin problems

There are many herbs which can be taken to alleviate the effects of certain skin disorders, such as red clover or figwort for psoriasis or yellow dock or burdock for eczema. Self-diagnosis, however, may not be sufficient in all cases. Contact dermatitis, for instance, may not need herbal treatment if the cause is an allergic reaction to some metal, such as nickel in your watch or jewellery. Likewise contact with an allergen such as grass or feathers may be causing the skin complaint.

Irritant eczema could be caused by a washing-up liquid or other detergent and can therefore be cleared up without the use of herbal remedies.

Not only would herbs be redundant in these cases, the treatment may mask the underlying need to rid yourself of the irritant or allergen.

Vomiting

Any sustained or prolonged vomiting should be treated professionally. Although herbs such as camomile and fennel can relieve nausea and vomiting, it is important that you rule out possible causes such as a perforated duodenal ulcer or gastroenteritis before you begin herbal treatment. Many digestive complaints are symptoms of other, more serious problems.

Chest pains

Mint or fennel may help to relieve the pain of indigestion but sudden chest pains may in fact be caused by muscular problems or be a precursor to a heart attack, in which case, seek immediate medical advice.

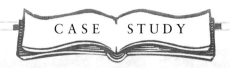

The Indigestion Sufferer

Self-treatment for persistent digestive problems without professional advice can be hazardous as many such pains may be symptoms of a serious disorder, such as colitis or appendicitis. If you have abdominal pain or indigestion which persists or is very uncomfortable it is vital that you seek medical attention to treat the underlying cause.

Tim is a 23-year-old legal secretary with a busy social life. He is careful with his weight, but tends to eat snacks and fast food. He has always had good health, apart from occasional constipation.

After two bouts of abdominal discomfort within a few weeks of each other, Tim thought he might have irritable bowel syndrome and decided to relax more and to cut down on fast foods. He also tried peppermint tea, which seemed to help. Tim had a further bout one evening, which was so bad he couldn't eat and had to lie down.

A recent episode was even worse, with extreme pain and a slight fever. This time he couldn't drink anything except water, and realised he would have to take further action.

WHAT SHOULD TIM DO?

Tim's attempts to improve his lifestyle and diet were both good ideas for general improvement in well-being, but his episodes of abdominal discomfort, which he attributed to an irritable bowel, were quite debilitating and recurrent, despite his attempts to deal with the problem. Ideally he should have sought professional help much sooner.

Taking peppermint tea is fine for symptomatic relief, but not as a substitute for correct diagnosis and treatment. If he had seen a doctor or practitioner straight away, it might have been possible to treat him promptly. Now that he has quite serious symptoms, Tim needs to call the doctor urgently.

Action Plan

HEALTH
Consult GP before symptoms become debilitating. Fast action can often provide a swift recovery.

SELF-HELP
Ensure a healthy, balanced diet and limit intake of fast foods from day to day to help to reduce the risk of major disorders.

LIFESTYLE
Take time to attend to illness properly. 'Quick-fix' remedies may lead to more serious complications.

HEALTH
Some serious medical problems can be masked by general symptoms and easily misdiagnosed.

SELF-HELP
Be aware that self-diagnosis and home treatment should not be continued if there is no sign of improvement within a day or so. This is most important if symptoms worsen.

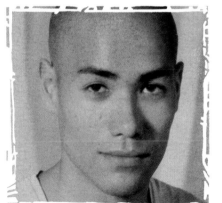

LIFESTYLE
Busy people often ignore signs of illness, but prolonged problems should be treated professionally.

HOW THINGS TURNED OUT FOR TIM

Tim called a friend, as he was beginning to feel very unwell. His friend was very worried by Tim's pains and called out the doctor, who examined Tim and diagnosed appendicitis. Tim's appendix was removed the next morning. Three weeks later he was out of hospital and back at work. Tim is still eating healthier foods, and goes to a yoga class for relaxation. The experience has made him much readier to seek professional help.

If you have an urgent condition that demands immediate medical attention, you should not take any form of herbal or self-help remedy, but seek immediate professional medical help, such as visiting your nearest Accident and Emergency department.

Symptoms such as severe loss of blood, breakages or fractures of bones should all be looked at immediately.

Likewise if you have received a heavy blow to the head, particularly if consciousness has been lost even if only for a few seconds, or you suffer unexplained drowsiness after such a blow, medical attention should be sought straight away.

Headaches

While feverfew, rosemary or camomile are good for soothing a headache, the real problem may be as simple as bad posture at work resulting in muscle strain in your neck. Correcting your seating position during the day could be all that is necessary to relieve your headaches. Likewise poor lighting when reading or unsuitable prescription glasses may be the cause of your headaches, and addressing those problems rather than just treating the symptoms makes the taking of herbs unnecessary. A persistent or worsening headache may be a sign of concussion, whilst a sharp pain in the head with pain behind the eyes may be caused by a brain tumour or stroke.

WHEN NOT TO USE HERBS

Some symptoms of serious illness demand immediate action. An understanding of the strengths and weaknesses of herbal remedies will help you to choose the most appropriate available treatment.

If your house catches fire you may experience severe nervous tension. You are, however, unlikely to take a remedy such as valerian, but rather try to put the fire out, or escape! Just the same, it is important to learn how to react to your medical symptoms in the most effective way in order to minimise any danger to your health. Although herbs are usually more gentle in their action than many of the analgesics and decongestants you can buy at your local chemist, they can still occasionally mask, or at least ameliorate, symptoms of serious illness. This is particularly true for digestive problems and some respiratory problems. It is therefore important to be aware of symptoms that may indicate serious trouble before using any form of self-medication.

PROTRACTED SYMPTOMS

There are certain symptoms that do not need to be brought immediately to the attention of a doctor, but if they persist for more than a few days, then you should seek help. These include: sudden weight loss without apparent cause; a constant thirst for no reason; having a mole increase in size or thickness, change colour or become itchy or bleed easily; a change in your voice – husky or hoarse; a change or lump in your breasts, nipples or scrotum; indigestion or acid belching; and feeling tired without good reason. Also the passing of blood whether in stools, urine, vomit or while coughing requires prompt attention.

OTHER SERIOUS SYMPTOMS

Apart from the above symptoms where medical treatment is imperative, there are some general rules to follow. If the problem is a familiar one which usually resolves itself – a chesty cough following a cold or a headache when tired, for example – use mild self-treatment and wait for it to pass.

Signs that you should seek professional help include: the failure of a mild condition to respond to herbal treatment within a reasonable period of time – generally a fortnight, but in feverish illnesses and other conditions such as continuous headaches, or headaches made worse by coughing, a week; a worsening of the condition; or the development of further symptoms.

Further to this, any sudden breathing problems, loss of vision, hearing or feeling, or the development of an exceptionally high temperature, should be treated as very serious and medical attention sought.

> **CAUTION**
> *Any medical complaints in children should be treated very seriously. Children are often less aware of the severity of their symptoms because they have little comparative experience.*
>
> *If a child becomes suddenly drowsy or has breathing problems, such as gulping, gasping for air, wheezing, or the inability to drink or speak, take them to the doctor straight away.*
>
> *A child who has pain on breathing in, violet spots that do not fade when pressed, weakness, drowsiness, confusion and does not react when spoken to should receive prompt medical attention. All of these symptoms are serious.*
>
> *Likewise severe diarrhoea and vomiting at the same time, and the inability to sit up or bend the head forward should be attended to immediately. Bleeding from any orifice and broken bones are, of course, medical emergencies.*

CHAPTER 4

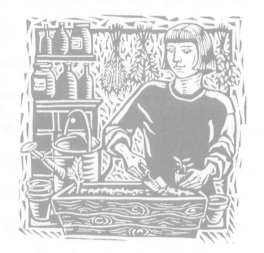

HERBAL PREPARATIONS

*Many professional herbalists still make their own
remedies, a tradition that has survived for centuries.
Commercially produced herbal medicines require
large-scale horticulture and complex manufacturing
processes with strict quality controls, but most herbs
can also be safely and successfully cultivated in pots
and gardens to be used as remedies at home.*

GROWING YOUR OWN HERBS

Anyone with a garden or a sunny windowsill can cultivate herbs. They are very self-sufficient plants and, given a little care and attention, will thrive almost anywhere.

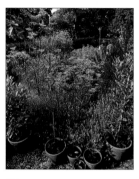

HERBS AT HOME
A herb garden need not overpower the rest of your garden. Set aside a small area just for your herbs, whether they are in pots or in beds. It may be most practical to plant your herbs near the house, especially the kitchen, so that you can tend and harvest them with ease.

The advantages of growing your own herbs are numerous. You do not need much space to create a herb garden – even a selection of herbs grown in a window box will provide a small annual harvest. Many herbs are very attractive and have culinary uses, so even if you do not wish to make medicines from them they will make a useful addition to your home.

GROWING YOUR OWN HERB GARDEN

Having your own herb garden gives you the opportunity to use the herbs immediately after they have been harvested, which can be important when making medical preparations at home. Growing culinary herbs in a flowerbed or in pots on a windowsill near the kitchen also makes them accessible and easy to tend, but choose a place away from busy streets and heavy traffic in order to avoid contamination by exhaust fumes.

Correct identification is absolutely essential when collecting plants for herbal remedies. Cutting the wrong herb for home use can at best make your medicine ineffective, but at worst it could lead to poisoning. If you grow your own herbs, buy seeds and seedlings from reputable suppliers so you will always know what you are planting and using. In addition, medicinal plants are becoming increasingly rare in the wild and most countries place restrictions on which plants may be picked. Growing your own supply of herbs, instead of gathering them, will help to preserve herbs growing in the

---

PLANNING A HERB GARDEN

Before you plant your herb garden, consider the space you have for your herbs and bear in mind which plants you want to grow.

Plot out your space and mark the areas that are best suited to your chosen plants. Identify the most sunny, shaded and moist areas of your garden and plant your herbs accordingly. If you are going to use your herbs frequently, make sure that you can reach them easily, without trampling other plants.

PLANNING YOUR GARDEN
Try to envisage how your garden will look once the plants have matured and how your herbs will work around fixed features such as trees and ponds.

Shady areas
Beds found around the base of trees and shadowed by walls or buildings are ideal for woodland herbs that thrive in partial sunlight. These include mint and lady's mantle.

Damp areas
Position water-loving plants such as bergamot and peppermint in any parts of your garden that naturally retain water, such as hollows or soil beside ponds.

Partial sun areas
Elecampane, marigold and borage are herbs that enjoy only partial sunlight. Areas that are shaded for parts of the day or that allow dappled light through are ideal.

Sunny areas
Most herbs adore bright sunshine and the sunniest area of your garden should contain your main herb bed. Plant herbs like hyssop and lavender here.

wild. If you take cuttings from plants make sure that you damage the plant as little as possible. When buying seeds, make sure they are dry and free from mould.

GETTING STARTED

Before you start planting, plan your herb garden carefully, taking into consideration space restrictions, the condition of the soil and which direction your garden faces.

Most herbs prefer a sunny, sheltered spot with well-drained soil but you should choose herbs that suit your particular garden. For warm, south-facing places choose sun-loving plants like thyme, rosemary and camomile and grow herbs like peppermint and marshmallow if your soil retains water.

Put tall plants like elecampane and mullein at the back of your border and let creepers such as thyme and lady's mantle spread along the border. If grown in the right conditions, herbs make few demands and need only a little basic care.

ANNUALS

Annual plants have to be grown from seed each spring. Herbs that belong to this group flower and produce seeds, and then die within their one-year life cycle. Most can be sown straight into the soil in mid or late spring. Some herbs, like parsley, germinate slowly and may need to be kept indoors until the seedlings are strong enough to be

GROWING HERBS IN POTS

Herbs look wonderful in containers, but do not like too much direct sunlight, because the heat makes them dry out quickly and saps their vitality. They need to be watered more often than their garden companions to keep them in good condition.

The key to success for healthy herbs in pots and window boxes lies in a good position, adequate drainage and a good quality potting compost. Choose a sunny but partially sheltered spot and make sure you plant the herbs in a container that accommodates them comfortably. Containers can also be easily moved indoors to give tender plants extra protection during the winter months.

Growing Herbs from Seeds and Cuttings

To ensure successful seed or root cultivation, make sure that seeds and roots are healthy and that any damage is kept to a minimum. Soil should be high quality, preferably loam-based, and should be kept moist. Any cuts to roots should be clean and neat, while seeds should be planted with adequate room for growth.

transferred to the garden soil. Annuals often do not grow very tall and can easily be planted among the perennials in your garden. Most of them are prolific seed producers and tend to self-seed – that is, they disperse their seeds themselves. They also make very good plants for window boxes and containers because many of them have attractive flowers. Easy-to-grow annuals include marigold and basil.

BIENNIALS

Biennials have a life cycle of two years, producing foliage in the first year and flowers and seeds in the second. Herbs in this category should be harvested in their second year, just before they die. They need to be sown again the following year. Biennial plants can grow quite tall, which you need to bear in mind when planning your herb garden. Among the herbs that belong to this group are angelica and cumin.

PERENNIALS

Perennial herbs will establish themselves and thrive for several years if grown in the right location. Some, like thyme and sage, are evergreen plants and keep their leaves during the winter months. Others, like feverfew and lady's mantle, die back in autumn to produce new growth each spring. Grow perennials in the largest bed in your garden and give them enough space to expand and reach their full size. Perennials have their own growing cycle, but unlike annuals or biennials, do not need to be replaced frequently. They will thrive for three to four years before they should be divided and replanted in a new location to give them enough room to keep them healthy. Cut back evergreen perennials each autumn to encourage vigorous growth the following year. Attractive perennials include wood betony, elecampane and juniper.

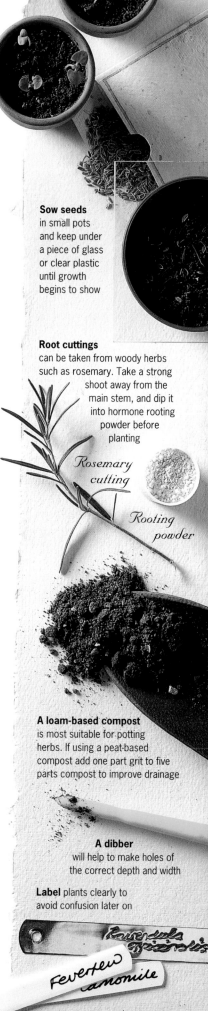

Sow seeds in small pots and keep under a piece of glass or clear plastic until growth begins to show

Root cuttings can be taken from woody herbs such as rosemary. Take a strong shoot away from the main stem, and dip it into hormone rooting powder before planting

Rosemary cutting

Rooting powder

A loam-based compost is most suitable for potting herbs. If using a peat-based compost add one part grit to five parts compost to improve drainage

A dibber will help to make holes of the correct depth and width

Label plants clearly to avoid confusion later on

The Horticulturist

Modern horticulture is the science of cultivating plants for both food and display. It includes the commercial growing of crops such as fruit, flowers and vegetables as well as all aspects of landscape gardening.

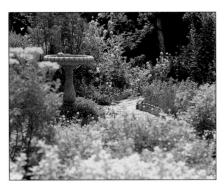

THE BEAUTY OF HERBS
Many herbs are cultivated for their beauty as well as their medicinal and culinary uses. Herbs have been an attractive feature in ornamental gardens for centuries.

THE HORTICULTURIST
Understanding the often astounding relationships between plants is a fundamental aspect of the horticulturist's trade. Planting French marigolds beside runner beans, for example, is a natural, organic way to control black fly.

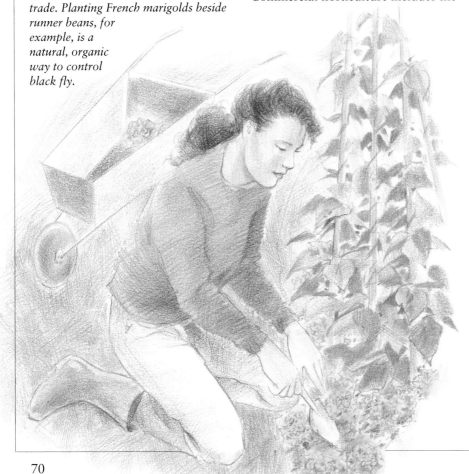

Modern horticulturists treat their vocation as a science and employ methods of propagating and harvesting plants that is way beyond what was known only a hundred years ago. However, traditional methods of growing crops are still used in organic horticulture, which is particularly important for the cultivation of medicinal plants.

What does horticulture involve?
Horticulture is divided into two areas: commercial and environmental. Commercial horticulture includes the large-scale growing and harvesting of crops such as fruits and vegetables for consumption as well as the cultivation of flowers for decorative purposes. This involves propagating the crop from seed, pricking out and potting up seedlings, and looking after them while they grow. Horticultural workers use fertilisers, pesticides and herbicides to obtain the maximum yield from their plants. The timing of a harvest is also very important in commercial horticulture as produce must be in peak condition when sold.

Environmental horticulture includes the planning, planting and maintenance of public and private gardens, parks and open spaces. Propagation and plant care are very similar to commercial horticulture, but harvesting is not an important part of the work, because the plants are not grown for consumption.

Do horticulturists grow herbs?
Many culinary herbs that are available in shops and garden centres have been grown by professional horticulturists using intensive cultivation methods – that is, fertilisers are used to make them grow faster in order to meet popular demand. In addition to this, they are treated routinely with herbicides and pesticides to keep them disease free. Herbs from such crops are acceptable for culinary use, but are not usually suitable for use as herbal medicines. Organically grown herbs are preferred for medicinal use because they carry no pesticide residues.

How are medicinal plants cultivated?
The best herbal preparations are made from plants that have been grown organically. Organic gardening is a relatively new branch of horticulture, but the methods organic gardeners use to grow their crops are based on very traditional and long-established practices.

In organic horticulture, plants are grown without the help of artificial fertilisers or disease control. Instead, organic gardeners take advantage of nature's ability to establish a healthy environment in which plants can thrive without the need for much intervention. This involves methods such as crop rotation, companion planting and biological pest control. Insects like ladybirds and hoverflies, for example, feed on certain common pests and so are welcomed as natural 'pesticides'. Crops are rotated frequently to keep the soil in good condition, which is important for healthy root growth. Organic horticulturists also know that certain plants grow well together while others do not and they plant their crops accordingly. Thus, for example, an organic horticulturist will know that the smell of onions deters the carrot fly and will therefore plant onions among carrots rather than use chemicals to preserve the crop.

Using these methods ensures that the herbal plants are able to develop their active constituents fully and are free from chemicals which might interfere with their healing powers.

Do organic horticulturists need special training?
Horticulture requires academic knowledge as well as a range of practical skills. Horticultural colleges teach sciences like biology and botany to give students a theoretical background, and also provide training in hands-on subjects such as crop management which involves propagation and harvesting. Many colleges also offer courses in organic horticulture to teach the specialist methods needed for this branch.

Origins

The cultivation of plants for food and medicine can be traced back thousands of years. Ancient civilisations like the Mayas of Central America and the Egyptians in Africa grew cereals for food, herbs for medicine and flowers for use in celebrations and rituals. Even then, the cultivation of plants was carefully planned and skilfully executed to get the best harvest possible.

In Britain, the spread of interest in horticulture grew from early settlements. The Middle Ages saw a vast interest in self-sufficiency coupled with an aesthetic pleasure in the beauty of gardens, and the Elizabethan gardens of the 16th century continue to influence the design of many public and private gardens today.

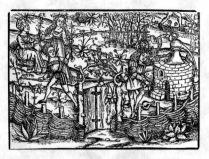

MEDIEVAL HERB GARDEN
The Middle Ages were an important time for horticulture in Europe. This period is famous for the kitchen and herb gardens of monasteries and royal palaces where plants were grown for culinary and medicinal purposes.

The scientific discoveries of the 20th century have shaped modern horticulture, which uses methods and techniques that allow plants to be cultivated on a much larger scale than before.

WHAT YOU CAN DO AT HOME

There are various methods of plant propagation that are easy to employ. Other than sowing seeds, two of the most popular techniques are to propagate from cuttings and by root division.

For the best cuttings, choose a healthy young plant and cut just below a leaf and stem joint with a clean, sharp knife. Try not to make more than one, clean cut. Dip the cut stem in a good-quality rooting preparation, which is widely available in nurseries and hardware shops. Insert the stem into compost and water well.

For propagation using root division, carefully divide a mature plant into smaller separate sections, ensuring that each section has a reasonable amount of root attached. Then simply replant the sections as individual plants.

ROOT DIVISION
It is important to use a clean, sharp knife when dividing roots and to ensure that damage to the root is minimal.

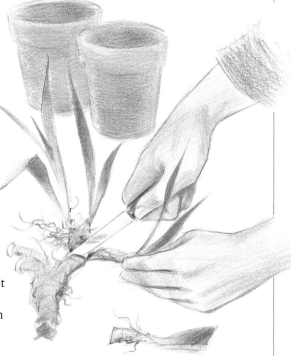

Herb Garden

Create a small herb garden on your balcony or windowsill by planting a few flowering pots or a culinary window box with easy-to-grow herbs such as basil, thyme and marigold.

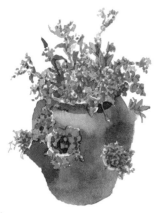

TERRACOTTA STRAWBERRY POT
Terracotta pots look beautiful but dry out quickly. Soak them in water several hours before planting to stop them taking moisture from newly potted plants.

Container planting allows you to move your herbs into sunlight or out of wind – even the smallest balcony can accommodate one or two pots. It is very important that you do not overcrowd the container because

herbs need ample 'leg room' for their roots. It is best to keep perennial herbs in individual pots. This will protect them during the winter, and will also prevent their roots from taking over the rest of the container.

PLANTING A WINDOW BOX

Window boxes made from plastic are very durable and retain moisture well, but do not have the same aesthetic appeal as terracotta. Other options include wooden troughs and painted tins.

To get started you will need your chosen window box, a good-quality loam-based potting compost and a selection of herbs. You will also need broken clay pots or pebbles for crocking;

these will allow the root system free drainage and air circulation. In effect, the crocking will ensure that you avoid waterlogging your container and so give your herbs a chance to mature.

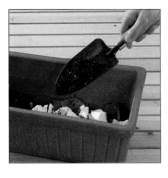

1 Cover the base of the container with 2.5 cm (1 in) of crocking material. Cover the crocks well with a layer of potting compost. Keep perennials in their pots to protect them when you replace your annuals when they die – plant annuals directly into the soil.

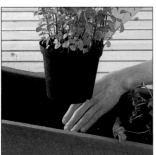

2 Place perennials with their pots in the container and fill the remaining space with compost to within 2.5 cm (1 in) of the rim. Always position tall plants at the back of the box.

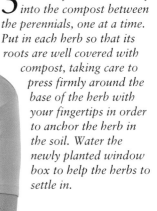

3 Plant any annuals directly into the compost between the perennials, one at a time. Put in each herb so that its roots are well covered with compost, taking care to press firmly around the base of the herb with your fingertips in order to anchor the herb in the soil. Water the newly planted window box to help the herbs to settle in.

CUTTING AND DRYING HERBS

All herbs have an optimum time when their leaves, flowers, seeds or roots should be harvested. To ensure the best herbal preparations, only harvest herbs at the recommended times.

Most herbs wilt soon after cutting and should be dried as soon as possible. Once dried, they should be kept in clean brown paper bags or dark glass containers away from direct sunlight. The most frequently used parts of a herb are its leaves, whether fresh or dried. The flowering parts can be used in many herbal preparations and the seeds are often used in spices or for drinks such as coffee and cocoa. Roots and tree bark are also sources of spices, such as ginger, and are used in the preparation of certain drugs, such as the malaria-countering quinine.

LEAVES
If you are preparing to make a herbal remedy using leaves, make sure you collect them on a dry day after the morning dew has evaporated. Aromatic herbs such as rosemary, sage and peppermint give off their fragrance, and with it their essential oils, in the midday sun and should be cut just before noon when their volatile oil content is at its highest.

Leaves are best harvested from young shoots, up to the time of flowering. Pick leaves from healthy plants which are free of dirt, disease or insect damage, taking care not to crush or bruise them.

Before drying, wipe off any soil, but do not wash the leaves as they are more likely to become mouldy if left damp. Cut herbs are very delicate and need to be kept out of direct sunlight as this will spoil their quality and diminish their therapeutic actions.

The best place to dry leaves is in a warm, dry, dark environment with reasonable ventilation. A drying temperature of around 24°C (75°F) is ideal. Most leaves will take about a week to dry completely, but very succulent or very thick leaves may take up to four. Spread the leaves thinly on paper (newspaper is not suitable as the printing ink may stain the leaves) or hang them up in small bunches and check them frequently. In fine weather, leaves may be dried outdoors in a sheltered, well-aired place, like a balcony or porch.

FLOWERS
Harvest flowers when their healing properties are at their best – just after they have opened. They should be picked in dry weather and before the midday heat. Choose undamaged flowers and pick them with great care, without bruising the petals if possible. After picking, keep the flowers out of direct sunlight and in a cool place, as they wilt very quickly.

Most flowers are very fragile and need to be handled carefully throughout the drying process. After cutting, spread them thinly on paper or muslin. Do not wash them as this would destroy all but the toughest flower heads. Flowers should retain their

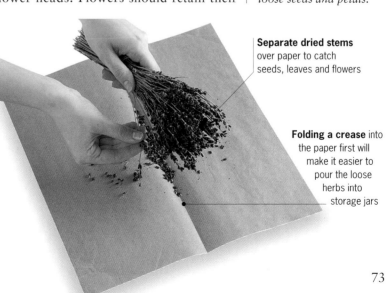

DRYING HERBS
A wire mesh stretched over a wooden frame makes an ideal drying rack, allowing air to circulate thoroughly. Alternatively, bunches of stems can be hung over a length of string or wooden rod in a warm place. Pack stems loosely to let air circulate. Cover flower heads with a bag while drying to catch loose seeds and petals.

Separate dried stems over paper to catch seeds, leaves and flowers

Folding a crease into the paper first will make it easier to pour the loose herbs into storage jars

colour if dried correctly but will fade if the temperature is too high. A room temperature of around 21°C (70°F) is generally ideal. Small flowers like camomile take about a week to dry, while larger flowers like marigolds can take up to three weeks to reach perfect dryness.

ROOTS

Roots should be collected in autumn, when the plant begins to store its therapeutic compounds below ground. Most roots that are used for medicinal purposes come from biennials or perennials and should be harvested in the plant's second or third year.

Dig up the roots carefully without crushing them or making unnecessary cuts. Decide how much you will need for yourself and replant the rest where you found it. Never take the whole root of perennials as this denies the plant the chance to regrow.

Most roots, such as dandelion and burdock, can be scrubbed clean with water before drying, but others like valerian should be cleaned gently with a damp cloth as their active principles are contained in the outer layer, which must be retained.

Cut large, thick roots lengthways into strips to aid drying. Roots dry better at higher temperatures than leaves or flowers

because they are more dense and tough. Between about 40–50°C (105–120°F) is ideal, but do not exceed a drying temperature of 60°C (140°F). Roots should be sliced before drying. They can be dried in an airing cupboard (two to five days) or in the oven with the door open (two to three hours), but need to be turned occasionally. The temperature is important but the flow of dry air is also a vital factor in drying. Check that your airing cupboard has an adequate airflow – the door should have holes or a gap in the bottom and top. When completely dry, roots will break easily in your hands.

SEEDS

Collect seeds when the seedpods of a plant are fully ripe. Ripe seed heads contain no green colour and have a papery texture. Always harvest seeds on a warm, dry day and shake them into a paper bag or onto a tray. Ripe seeds should come off the heads easily. Make sure you save some of the seeds from annual plants for propagation to ensure a good harvest the following year.

Seeds dry very quickly in airy, warm conditions, such as an airing cupboard: they will be ready for storage after a week or two. The temperature for drying seeds is the same as for roots, but it is not advisable to dry seeds in the oven. Many seeds are collected for their aromatic properties and drying at too high a temperature will evaporate the aromatic oils.

BARKS

The best time to collect the bark of trees is in damp weather, since it peels off more easily when wet than when dry. Take the fresh bark from young trunks or branches, but never take a whole ring of bark from around the tree's girth as this may interfere with its feeding system and may also cause irreparable damage.

Check the stripped bark for insects and moss and remove them carefully with a damp cloth. Bark will dry more quickly in small pieces than in one large section. Dry bark in a warm, dark and airy place at the same temperature as for roots (around 50°C or 120°F) until the bark feels dry and breaks easily. This may take anything from one to four weeks.

Barks can be dried in the oven, again at the same temperature as roots: 40–50°C (105–120°F). Drying will take 2–3 hours.

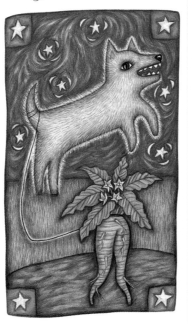

Herbal Myths

Mandrake, with its human-shaped root, is regarded in legend to be an aphrodisiac and virility boost, and has long been considered a supernatural being. The being was believed to emit a scream on uprooting so chilling and powerful that it could kill the harvester.

To avoid such a death, harvesters would tie a dog to the root by its tail and let the dog suffer the screams. Uprooting was carried out at night to protect the power of the root and this no doubt added to the superstitious myths surrounding the plant.

TYPES OF PREPARATION

Herbs can be used in so many ways, it is important to have some understanding of the different types of preparation that are possible when choosing or making a herbal remedy.

Once you are aware of the different properties of herbs you can decide on the best preparation for your needs. Some preparations require time and special materials, whilst others simply need boiling water. Thorough sterilisation of all utensils is very important when preparing herbal remedies. Sterilising your equipment for 30 minutes before use will help to ensure that your preparations are free of germs and will lengthen the life of creams and syrups as they will be less likely to become mouldy.

When choosing a remedy it is very important to consider both the ailment that you are going to treat (see Chapter 6) and the parts of herb or herbs that you are intending to use (see Chapter 5).

INTERNAL PREPARATIONS
Most preparations for internal use are liquids that have the active ingredients of the herbs drawn into the solution. Whether water or alcohol-based, liquid internal preparations are among the simplest herbal remedies to make and require little or no special equipment.

Infusions
Also called teas or tisanes, infusions are water-based extracts of plants, recommended for preparing the delicate parts of a plant, such as the flowers, leaves and green stems. They are notably used where a mild preparation is required, for example for children or those who cannot tolerate alcohol. Infusions are also used for compresses and where a mild external application is desired.

Hot infusions are made with water that has been boiled then left to stand for 30 seconds. Use 25 g (1 oz) of dried herb or 50 g (1¾ oz) of fresh herb to make 600 ml (1 pint) of tea. Put the herb into a warmed china or glass teapot – not a metal one – and pour the hot water over it. Cover and steep for

EQUIPMENT
Some preparations have clearly defined steps, just like recipes, so it is always best to have all the equipment that you are going to need to hand before you begin. Some quick remedies, such as inhalations, are easy to prepare but may become unusable if left to cool while you search for a towel to cover your head.

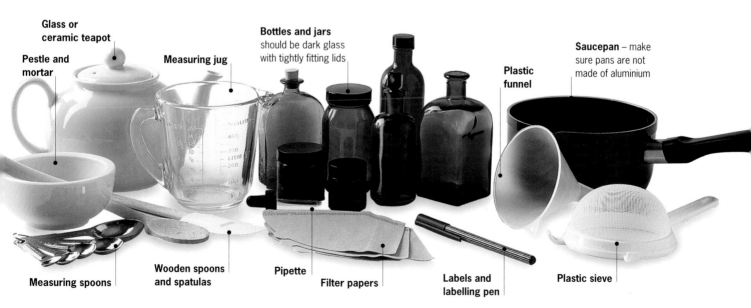

Glass or ceramic teapot

Pestle and mortar

Measuring jug

Bottles and jars should be dark glass with tightly fitting lids

Plastic funnel

Saucepan – make sure pans are not made of aluminium

Measuring spoons

Wooden spoons and spatulas

Pipette

Filter papers

Labels and labelling pen

Plastic sieve

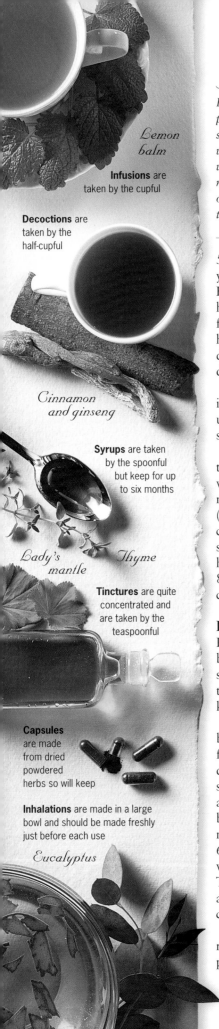

Infusions are taken by the cupful

Lemon balm

Decoctions are taken by the half-cupful

Cinnamon and ginseng

Syrups are taken by the spoonful but keep for up to six months

Lady's mantle   *Thyme*

Tinctures are quite concentrated and are taken by the teaspoonful

Capsules are made from dried powdered herbs so will keep

Inhalations are made in a large bowl and should be made freshly just before each use

Eucalyptus

Herbal Preparations

Both internal preparations (left) and external preparations (see far right) are tailored to treat specific ailments and as such must be prepared very carefully. It is a good idea to be able to visualise your preparation to know how much to make and to take. An infusion, for example, is often the size of a cup of tea, while tinctures are taken by the teaspoonful.

5–10 minutes, depending on the strength you require. Strain and sip slowly while hot. Herbal infusions may be sweetened with honey or brown sugar, or flavoured with fresh lemon juice. The standard dosage for herbal teas is one cup two or three times a day for adults, and half this amount for children under 12, unless stated otherwise.

Infusions should be prepared and used immediately. They can be refrigerated for up to two days, but if there is any sign of spoiling, an infusion must be discarded.

Some plants contain active constituents that are water soluble, but are destroyed when heated. Herbs like marshmallow or mullein contain large amounts of mucilage (see page 84) and need to be prepared as cold infusions. The quantities for cold infusions are the same as for hot teas. Soak the herb in cold water in a glass or china pot for 8–12 hours (or overnight); strain and drink cold. Prepare fresh every day.

Decoctions

Like infusions, decoctions are water-based, but are used for the tough parts of the herbs, such as seeds, barks and roots, that release their active constituents only if cut or broken into small pieces and simmered.

To prepare a decoction use 25 g (1 oz) broken dried herb or 50 g (1¾ oz) chopped fresh herb to make 600 ml (1 pint) of the decoction. Put the herb into an enamel or stainless-steel pan, cover with cold water and a tight-fitting lid. Slowly bring to the boil, then reduce the heat and simmer for 15 minutes. Strain and add water to make up 600 ml (1 pint) if necessary. Sip slowly while hot and sweeten with honey if desired. The standard dose is half a cup three times a day for adults and half this amount for children under 12, unless stated otherwise.

Decoctions will keep for three days if refrigerated, but are at their most effective if prepared fresh every day.

Tinctures

Tinctures are alcohol-based extracts of plants and are much stronger than teas or decoctions so are taken in much smaller doses. For many plant constituents alcohol is a better solvent than water because it can extract a wider range of plant chemicals. It concentrates the remedy and also acts as a preservative – stored correctly, tinctures will keep for up to three years.

Tinctures can be made from fresh or dried herbs depending on the availability of the plants. When tinctures are produced professionally, specific water-to-alcohol proportions are used for each herb, but for home use diluted vodka makes an excellent base.

Put 225 g (8 oz) of cut dried herb or 450 g (1 lb) of the fresh plant into a large jar. Pour 700 ml (1¼ pints) of vodka and 300 ml (½ pint) of water over the herb and close the jar tightly. Keep the container in a warm place for two weeks, shaking it well once a day. Strain off the liquid through a muslin cloth suspended over a bowl. Squeeze the remaining liquid from the solid residue into the bowl, then discard the solids.

Pour the tincture into a dark glass bottle and label with the herb used and the date it was made. It is now ready to use. Keep in a cool place away from direct sunlight.

A standard dose for a tincture is between 5–20 drops or up to 5 ml (1 teaspoon) three times a day for adults. Children under 12 should take 5–10 drops or up to 2.5 ml (½ teaspoon) three times a day. They can be taken neat or mixed with a little water. Mixing the drops of tincture with hot water will allow the alcohol to evaporate and leave only the herbal extract to be taken.

Syrups

Syrups are the traditional way of making medicines palatable for children. Sugar-based preparations also help to soothe and protect irritated and inflamed body tissue. The standard dosage for adults is 10 ml (2 teaspoons) three times a day; children should take 5 ml (1 teaspoon) three or four times a day, unless stated otherwise by a doctor or herbalist.

To make 1 litre (1¾ pints) of syrup, you need 225 g (8 oz) of dried herb or 450 g (1 lb) of fresh herbs, 2 litres (3½ pints) of filtered or bottled water and 900 g (2 lb) of caster sugar. Bring the water to the boil then stir in the herb and simmer gently over a low heat for 10 minutes. Strain the decoction through a muslin cloth, taking care to squeeze all the liquid from the solid residue. Transfer the decoction into a bain marie and reduce slowly to 500 ml (18 fl oz). This will take about two hours. Add the sugar and stir over a gentle heat until the sugar has completely dissolved. Be careful not to let the sugar boil or burn.

When the syrup is cool, pour into a dark glass bottle, label and store in a cool place. Syrups should be used within six months.

Capsules

Powdered herbs can be sprinkled on food or taken with water, but are most easily taken as capsules. Capsule cases and powdered herbs are available from herbal suppliers.

To prepare capsules, pour the powder into a saucer and slide the capsule halves through the powder. When they are full, join the halves together to seal the capsule.

Inhalants

Inhalants or vapours are preparations that contain large amounts of volatile oils. They are used to relieve congestion, inflammation and infections of the airways (see page 78).

EXTERNAL PREPARATIONS

Preparations for external use mainly comprise the active herb ingredients in a form that most readily applies the therapeutic qualities to the affected area. These include poultices, creams and lotions.

Essential or volatile oils are sometimes used instead of the solid herb. These are added to base oils, creams or wax and make preparation easier.

Compresses

Water-based herbal preparations that are applied directly to the skin with a cloth are called compresses. Because these can be prepared and applied quickly to the affected

Sage

Herb oils keep for months in a jar with an airtight lid

Creams can be used liberally and keep well

Mallow and rose

Ointments are used on small areas only but can be stored

Marigold

Lotions should be prepared fresh each time

Eyebright

Liniments are used sparingly so a little goes a long way

Cayenne pepper

Compresses are made by soaking a clean piece of cloth in a freshly prepared decoction or infusion

Poultices are made to cover a specific area. You need only enough to repeat the treatment two or three times

---

MAKING COMPRESSES AND POULTICES

Compresses can be applied hot or cold, depending on the conditions they are used for. Cold compresses are applied when the skin feels hot to the touch, in such cases as inflammations, hot joints and swellings. Hot compresses are useful to relieve cramps and muscle tension. Poultices are mainly used to draw pus from the skin, heal abscesses and boils and draw splinters. You should prepare sufficient amounts of the herb to cover the affected area.

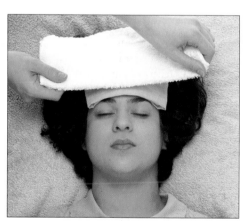

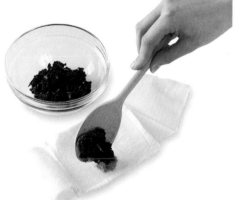

COMPRESSES
To make a compress, soak a clean cotton cloth in a herbal infusion or decoction, place it over the affected part and cover with a clean towel. Keep replacing the compress to keep the area cool or hot as required. For cold compresses cool the liquid before use by making a strong infusion or decoction and adding ice cubes after straining the liquid.

POULTICES
For a poultice, dried or powdered herbs must be mixed to a paste with hot water and spread onto clean gauze before application to the skin. Drop some linseed or olive oil on the area to be covered as this will make removal of the poultice easier. Cover with a cotton cloth and keep in place until the poultice has cooled. Repeat as necessary.

Inhalants

Inhalants relieve nasal congestion and help to fight sinus infections. They can be made as aromatic rubs for longer-term inhalation, or you can inhale the steam from infused herbs for immediate symptom relief.

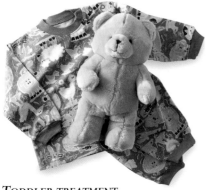

TODDLER TREATMENT
Children often find the discomfort of blocked airways distressing. This distress may be lessened with a few drops of essential oil on your child's bedding or teddy to help him or her settle to a comfortable night's sleep.

For an instant inhalant to relieve congestion from hay fever or colds, blend a selection of essential oils and dab them onto a handkerchief or place on a pillowcase, then inhale. Inhalants are particularly effective for night-time relief. Because most essential oils are powerful, concentrated preparations, they should be taken only in very small quantities and used for the short-term relief of acute symptoms.

Essential oils like eucalyptus, pine, peppermint and cajeput have long been known as effective decongestants and antiseptic remedies for all sorts of sinus problems. Blended oils can be inhaled directly.

MAKING YOUR OWN VAPOUR RUB

To prepare your own rub, use Vaseline as a base and add essential oils to it. Vaseline is not absorbed by the skin, but acts as a carrier for the oils and lets them evaporate when massaged into the chest. Inhaling the vapours takes the oils' healing properties directly to the airways to soothe inflamed sinuses and act as decongestants. Used sparingly it is also suitable for infants and children. Stored in a cool, dark place the mixture will keep for up to a year.

Equipment
China or stainless-steel bowl
Wooden spoon or spatula
Saucepan
Small measuring jug
Dark glass jar (50 ml, 2 fl oz) or, if you prefer, two small dark glass jars (30 ml, 1 fl oz)
Labels

Ingredients
5 tbsp Vaseline
20 drops peppermint oil
20 drops eucalyptus oil
20 drops cajeput oil
5 drops pine oil

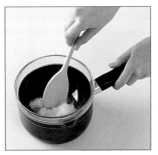

1 *Put the Vaseline in the bowl and suspend it over a saucepan which has been filled with enough water to cover the bottom. Slowly heat until the Vaseline has just melted.*

2 *Remove from the heat and transfer the Vaseline to a small measuring jug. Leave to cool for 2 minutes, stirring continuously.*

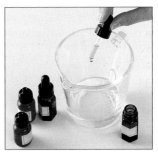

3 *Add the essential oils drop by drop, continuing to stir.*

4 *Pour the mixture into the jars. Leave to cool further and seal when the mixture has reached room temperature. Label each jar with the name and date.*

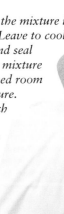

NIGHT-TIME RELIEF
Massaging vapour rub into your chest before you go to sleep will ensure that you inhale the decongestant vapours all night and wake breathing freely.

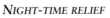

area, hot and cold compresses are ideal for relieving bruising, swelling, headaches and many sporting injuries.

Whether used hot or cold, for the best results compresses should be soaked and reapplied frequently.

Poultices

Simmered warm herbs that are applied directly to the skin and held in place with a dressing are called poultices. The heat and active ingredients in a poultice make it ideal for infections and muscular pain. Poultices used to be a favourite remedy for skin infection such as boils.

Creams

Creams are light, nourishing preparations that spread easily and are absorbed into the skin. They contain natural waxes, oils and a non-oily substance such as a tincture or a floral water. Creams are very useful for treating conditions that can affect large areas of the body, for example dry skin, psoriasis and eczema. Creams are particularly effective for treating conditions that need moisturising, such as patches of rough, chapped or dry skin. The cream forms a protective layer to reduce further complications and the active herbal ingredients help to soothe the skin and treat the underlying disorder.

Ointments

Ointments are much thicker than creams, because they consist of waxes and oils only, rather than a mixture of oil and water. They do not penetrate the skin very well and act more as a protective barrier against infection and external factors. Use ointments for conditions that cover only a small area of skin such as cuts, grazes and small patches of psoriasis. Underlying conditions that cause such skin problems may need other applications to combat the disorder, but ointments will help to relieve symptoms and

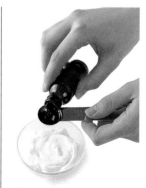

A SIMPLE CREAM
The easiest way to make a cream is to add a tincture or essential oil to a base cream. Add 20 ml (⅔ fl oz) of tincture to 50 ml (2 fl oz) of unscented base cream (available from chemists). For essential oils add 8 drops to 50 ml (2 fl oz) cream.

MAKING CREAMS AND OINTMENTS

To prepare a cream from basic ingredients involves creating an emulsion between water and an oil or fat. The process must be carried out carefully to avoid separation. Once made, creams must be refrigerated or stored in airtight jars to keep them fresh. Unlike creams, ointments contain no water and are prepared with a base of petroleum jelly, beeswax or paraffin wax. The consistency of the ointment can be altered to suit the application – the more solid the ointment the less oily it will be.

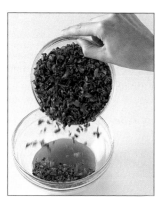 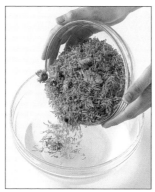 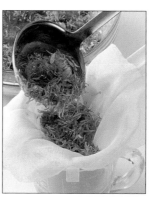 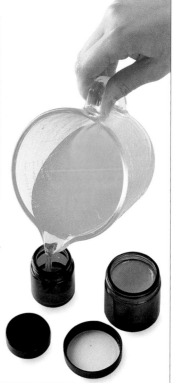

MAKING A CREAM
To make a cream, melt 175 g (6 oz) emulsifying wax (available from chemists) in a bowl over a pan of boiling water. Remove from the pan and stir in 25 g (1 oz) dried herb, 75 g (2¾ oz) glycerine and 75 ml (2½ fl oz) water. Return to the pan and simmer for three hours.

MAKING AN OINTMENT
Melt 450 g (1 lb) petroleum jelly or paraffin wax in a bowl over a pan of boiling water. Remove from the heat then stir in 55 g (2 oz) finely chopped dried herb. Return to the pan and simmer for 15 minutes, stirring all the time.

1 *For both preparations, strain the hot mixture through a jelly bag or a piece of muslin laid over a sieve. Squeeze out excess liquid.*

2 *Cool slightly, then pour the still soft mixture into sterilised dark glass jars and leave to set. When cool, secure lids, label and store.*

speed recovery. If symptoms persist seek the advice of a qualified practitioner. It is possible that the action of the ointment may mask the signs of a serious problem.

Liniments

Liniments are oily preparations designed to be easily absorbed through the skin to stimulate blood flow underneath. Very hot spices like cayenne pepper, for example, are traditional ingredients in a liniment. The skin will become very red and hot after application as the blood flow increases under the surface of the skin. This increased flow helps to heal injury and infection.

MAKING LINIMENTS AND LOTIONS

Liniments are powerful healing tools for the pain of arthritic conditions and diseases of the airways, but should never be used on broken skin because rubefacient herbs will irritate.

Floral waters like rose or camomile water are good examples of skin lotions. They should be dabbed onto the skin with clean cotton wool or other absorbent fabric.

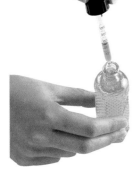

TO MAKE A LINIMENT
Mix one part of infused herb oil (see right) with an equal part of tincture, bottle and label. For every 100 ml (3½ fl oz) of the mixture you may add up to 10 drops of essential oils. A liniment will keep indefinitely and should be very well shaken before use. Massage gently into the skin, taking care to wash your hands afterwards. Repeat as necessary.

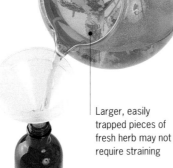

Larger, easily trapped pieces of fresh herb may not require straining

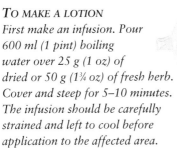

TO MAKE A LOTION
First make an infusion. Pour 600 ml (1 pint) boiling water over 25 g (1 oz) of dried or 50 g (1¾ oz) of fresh herb. Cover and steep for 5–10 minutes. The infusion should be carefully strained and left to cool before application to the affected area.

Lotions

Lotions are also liquid preparations for external use, but unlike liniments contain little or no oily substances. They can be applied directly to the skin, such as with a compress, or used as washes for eyes, ears and mouth. To make an eye lotion, make a standard infusion, add a pinch of salt and strain through a fine filter (coffee filters are ideal). Use with an eye bath from the chemist or as a compress twice a day. Make a fresh infusion for each application and make sure the infusion is clear of any solids – you may exacerbate the problem if small pieces of herb get into your eyes. Use fresh lotion for each eye to avoid cross-infection.

Infused herb oils

Unlike essential oils, infused herb oils are stable preparations and therefore they do not evaporate, even when heated. Infused oils are particularly useful as massage oils and are important ingredients for many ointments, rubs and liniments.

To make an infused oil, fill a clear glass jar with fresh herbs and cover them with a light vegetable oil; sunflower, grapeseed or almond are suitable. Close the jar tightly and leave to stand in a warm, sunny place for four to six weeks. Strain through a muslin cloth into a dark bottle, label and date. Stored in a cool, dark place it will keep for several months.

Other herbal preparations

Aside from the most popular and common uses, many herbal remedies can be tailored to more specific preparations to treat various disorders.

Gargles and mouthwashes made from sage and thyme infusions are ideal for relieving sore throats and mouth ulcers. Try to use gargles as hot as possible to get the best effects.

Juices are simple to make and are easily applied externally or taken internally. A juice extractor, available from kitchen shops, makes juicing easy.

Plaisters are cloth strips impregnated with wax and essential oils. These are applied externally and, as the body's heat softens the wax, the essential oils are released.

Pessaries and suppositories may be recommended by your herbalist. It is probably safest to buy ready-made pessaries and suppositories from your herbalist.

HERBS IN YOUR DIET

Many popular culinary herbs have disinfecting and antioxidant properties which help to preserve foods, especially meat, as well as aiding the digestive system in breaking down food.

Using herbs for cooking is different from taking them medicinally. The amounts are usually smaller and heating the herb in cooking usually lessens its medicinal effect. Nevertheless, herbs in the diet can stimulate appetite and digestion and ease the symptoms of trapped wind. The culinary use of herbs is firmly recommended alongside other treatments for lack of appetite or difficulty in digesting food.

INTRODUCING HERBS TO YOUR FOOD

Most of the herbs we eat have very mild effects, and to overeat any of them would take a deliberate and serious effort. If the herb completely overwhelms the taste of the food, that is overdoing it. Spices can irritate or overstimulate a sensitive digestive system, and if you have gastritis, a peptic ulcer or irritable bowel syndrome you should avoid pepper and cayenne, for example, although ginger may well be helpful. Large amounts of cayenne and rosemary should be avoided if you suffer from raised blood pressure.

Cooking can have an effect on the medicinal properties of the herb. For example, cooking degrades the antibacterial substances in garlic but does not affect its cardiovascular properties (see page 89). Most of the volatile oils of many culinary herbs are lost during cooking, so that their anti-infective properties are greatly diminished. To preserve these, herbs can be added to a dish after it has been taken off the heat.

Fresh, aromatic herbs are usually more stimulating than dried herbs, but with good quality dried herbs the difference is less noticeable after prolonged cooking. The antibacterial and circulatory properties of ginger (see page 132) are, however, more powerful after drying. Some herbs, such as parsley and basil, taste far better when fresh.

HERBAL FEASTS
Many herbs make wonderful additions to everyday and exotic dishes. A herb salad is a delicious way of boosting your intake of herbs and benefiting from their therapeutic actions.

HERBAL TEAS

Culinary herbs need not only be used for cooking, they can also be used as the basis for a refreshing, soothing, invigorating or calming cup of tea.

Particularly effective culinary herbs for making tea include thyme, mint, lemon balm and fennel. Non-culinary herbs that make great tea include hops, rosehip, hibiscus, camomile, lemon verbena, meadowsweet or skullcap.

For a refreshing and invigorating tea, use blackberry or blackcurrant leaves, rosemary, nettle or peppermint. If you want a soothing and relaxing cup, after an exhausting day at work for example, use aniseed, basil, fennel or marjoram.

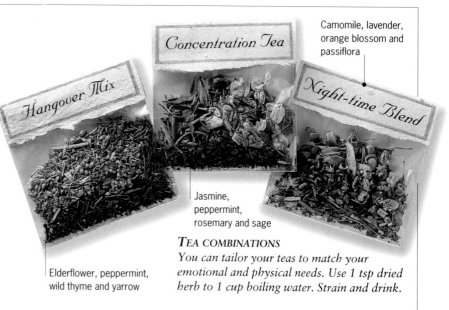

Camomile, lavender, orange blossom and passiflora

Jasmine, peppermint, rosemary and sage

Elderflower, peppermint, wild thyme and yarrow

TEA COMBINATIONS
You can tailor your teas to match your emotional and physical needs. Use 1 tsp dried herb to 1 cup boiling water. Strain and drink.

WHICH HERBS FOR WHICH FOODS

The following selection of everyday culinary herbs are all suitable for using fresh or dried, chopped, ground, grated or powdered when cooking.

Although many of the herbs below are well known and recommended for certain foods or dishes there is no reason not to experiment by adding your favourite herbs to any dishes you prepare. Wilting the leaves by quickly frying them in a hot dressing offers an alternative presentation. They will also help, to some extent, to soothe or relieve a particular ailment, or they may simply be used to intensify the flavour, add spice or make your food look more interesting.

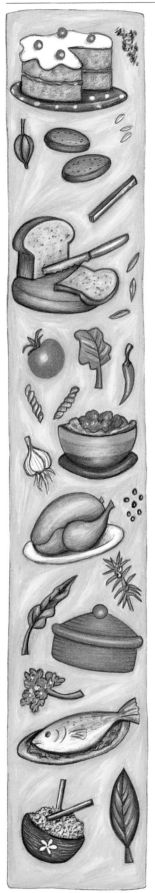

HERB	CULINARY USE	THERAPEUTIC ACTION
Aniseed	Can be used in the baking of cakes, making sweets and savouries and in tomato-based sauces	An appetite stimulant, helps to expel trapped wind and is a relaxing expectorant
Angelica	Chop leaves for vegetable salads or court bouillon for seafood	Aids indigestion, relieves constipation and freshens bad breath
Basil	Along with garlic, this makes an excellent pesto sauce. Also good with Mediterranean dishes and rice salads	Clears the head and sinuses and helps to expel trapped wind
Bay	Use in a bouquet garni, and in soups, casseroles and with rice	Expels trapped wind
Black pepper	Can be used to season almost anything from soups to curries to pasta dishes	An aromatic digestive stimulant, helps to expel trapped wind
Caraway	Sprinkle onto rich meats, or to flavour soups and breads	Calming to the digestion and helps to expel trapped wind
Cardamom	Enhances sweet and savoury dishes especially in Indian cooking	Expels trapped wind and relieves indigestion and headaches
Cayenne pepper	Sprinkle onto rich meats, or use to flavour soups, breads and cakes	A powerful digestive and circulatory stimulant, relieves stomach pains and cramp
Celery seeds	Used to enhance the flavour of soups, stews or omelettes	A digestive stimulant, helps to expel trapped wind and is a cleansing diuretic
Cinnamon	Flavours stews and goes well with any apple dish, especially cakes	Is antiseptic and warming
Coriander	Add fresh leaves to enhance soups. Mix into stews and curries	Is aromatic, disinfecting and helps to expel trapped wind
Dandelion	Add fresh leaves to salads	Is diuretic and cleansing
Fennel	Flavours chicken, fish and pork. Chop leaves for a tasty addition to salads	An aromatic digestive stimulant, expectorant and antidepressant and helps to expel trapped wind
Garlic	Goes well with sauces, meat dishes, casseroles, dressings, patés and dips	Anti-inflammatory, anti-infective, stimulates digestion and promotes cardiovascular health
Marjoram (Oregano)	Add fresh to Italian dishes, salad dressings and grilled meats	A warming digestive and circulatory stimulant
Parsley	Chop into fish, rice and pasta dishes	Is disinfecting, cleansing and diuretic
Rosemary	Use fresh in salads or to flavour pork and lamb dishes	A warming digestive and circulatory stimulant, for depression, fatigue, rheumatic pains, enhancing concentration and memory
Sage	Use in stuffings or cook with strong-flavoured meats	An antiseptic and digestive stimulant, good for menopausal problems and diarrhoea
Thyme	Adds flavour to meat stews, soups, tomato-based sauces or roast poultry	A disinfectant and expectorant, it also helps to relieve digestive problems
Turmeric	Used in curries, add to fish, poultry and vegetables	Anti-inflammatory and soothing to the digestion

CHAPTER 5

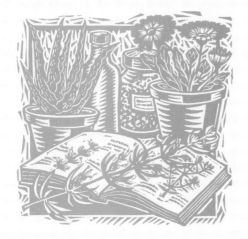

A GUIDE TO THE HEALING HERBS

To decide between a tincture of rosehips and a camomile poultice, to find yarrow growing in the wild or to know what to look for when harvesting goldenseal requires knowledge that has been refined over thousands of years. This chapter puts this knowledge at your fingertips and gives a valuable insight into the art of herbalism.

CHOOSING HERBAL REMEDIES

The active constituents of different herbs coupled with the various methods of preparation available can give valuable guidelines to the most effective remedies for health problems.

Reading the recommended doses
In general, tinctures are noted as having a ratio, for example 1:5, which means that for every 1 part herb you should add 5 parts liquid. This liquid will contain a percentage of alcohol, for example 12%, which should form the base of the liquid (see page 76). Finally, a recommended dose is given in millilitres. All doses for infusions are for dried herbs – you should double the given amount if you are using fresh herbs. Each dose is per cup. All the remedies should be taken three times a day, unless otherwise stated.

In this chapter you will find a selection of popular herbs and their recommended medicinal uses. For each herb there is a description of its physical characteristics, a guide to where it is commonly found and, where relevant, some historical and background information.

There is also a description of the actions of the herbs, definitions of which are given in more detail in Chapter 3 (see pages 53–55), and their best-known and most widely applied uses.

This is followed by recommended preparations and dosages. Details of the methods of preparation are given in Chapter 4. Each entry concludes with any known cautions and contraindications.

CHEMICALS AND COMPOUNDS

The active constituents of a herb are the chemicals and compounds it contains which act on other substances. The various constituents are grouped according to their actions or chemical make-up.

Herbs rich in alkaloids usually have strong pharmaceutical actions such as the stimulants that are found in caffeine and in capsaicin from chilli peppers.

Anthraquinones are laxative. They stimulate the bowel after being absorbed into the system – hence their delayed action. Senna and rhubarb root contain anthraquinones.

Bitters are a varied group of constituents linked by their bitter taste. The bitterness stimulates the salivary glands and digestive organs, which improves appetite and digestion. Gentian and wormwood are bitters.

Coumarins, on the other hand, are aromatic substances, often used in perfumery. In the body they act as carminatives, antidepressants and antiseptics. In pharmacology they are used as anticoagulants – they help to thin the blood. Herbs that contain coumarins include angelica and red clover.

Flavonoids also improve circulation by strengthening blood vessels and are often anti-inflammatory. Flavonoid-rich herbs include hawthorn and yarrow.

Mucilage and gums are viscous substances found in plants, made up of molecules of complex sugars (polysaccharides). The sugar molecules soak up water to form a soft, jelly-like substance which coats the lining of the digestive tract with a soothing, sticky, protective layer. The soothing action extends to the lungs and bladder. Soothing herbs with a high mucilage content include marshmallow and fenugreek.

Resins are liquids from the stems of plants. With their antiseptic and antifungal actions, resins stimulate the immune system to fight infection. Echinacea and marigold are notable resinous herbs.

Tannins dry and contract the body's tissues, drawing them together and improving their resistance to infection. Herbs rich in tannins include tea and cinnamon.

Although antiseptic and soothing when taken internally, phenolic acids can be very irritating when applied directly to the skin. Salicylic acid, the forerunner of aspirin, is one of the best-known phenols.

Antiarthritic herbs such as meadowsweet, contain soothing, analgesic salicylates. Aspirin was originally made from meadowsweet, but unlike aspirin, meadowsweet in its natural form does not upset the digestion.

The word saponin derives from *sapo*, which is Latin for soap. Like soap, saponins dissolve fats and can alter the balance of hormones in the body. Herbs rich in saponins include wild yam and ginseng.

LINNAEUS' HERBAL CLASSIFICATION

The herbs in this chapter are listed in alphabetical order under their Latin rather than their common name. The classification system using Latin names was originated by the Swedish botanist Carolus Linnaeus (Carl von Linné) (1707-1778) and has been used ever since as the most comprehensive and precise method of classifying plants. The Latin names will help you to ensure that you have exactly the right plant for your needs – not one that merely looks similar, is from the same family or has a similar common name. In many cases the difference can be vital – neroli oil, for example, only comes from the bitter orange plant, not from all orange plants, so accuracy is important. On the other hand, some plant species, such as aloes, all contain the necessary active ingredients. In these cases you will find the most common variety listed.

COMMON NAME	LATIN NAME	COMMON NAME	LATIN NAME	COMMON NAME	LATIN NAME
Agnus castus	Vitex agnus-castus	Fennel	Foeniculum vulgare	Onion	Allium cepa
Agrimony	Agrimonia eupatoria	Fenugreek	Trigonella foenum-graecum	Oregon grape	Mahonia aquifolium
Aloe vera	Aloe vera	Feverfew	Tanacetum parthenium	Parsley	Petroselinum crispum
Angelica	Angelica archangelica	Figwort	Scrophularia nodosa	Passionflower	Passiflora incarnata
Apple	Malus spp.	Galangal	Alpinia officinarum	Peppermint	Mentha x piperita
Barley	Hordeum vulgare	Garlic	Allium sativum	Plantain (psyllium)	Plantago spp.
Basil	Ocimum basilicum	Gentian	Gentiana lutea	Pokeroot	Phytolacca americana
Bay	Laurus nobilis	Ginger	Zingiber officinalis	Raspberry	Rubus idaeus
Betony	Stachys officinalis	Goldenseal	Hydrastis canadensis	Red clover	Trifolium pratense
Bilberry	Vaccinium myrtillus	Hawthorn	Cratageus oxyacantha	Rose	Rosa spp.
Bitter orange	Citrus aurantium	Hops	Humulus lupulus	Rosemary	Rosmarinus officinalis
Black haw	Viburnum prunifolium	Horse chestnut	Aesculus hippocastanum	Sage	Salvia officinalis
Bladderwrack	Fucus vesiculosus	Horsetail	Equisetum arvense	Skullcap	Scutellaria spp.
Borage	Borago officinalis	Hyssop	Hyssopus officinalis	Sea holly	Eryngium maritimum
Burdock	Arctium lappa	Juniper	Juniperus communis	Shepherd's purse	Capsella bursa-pastoris
Camomile	Chamomilla recutita	Lady's mantle	Alchemilla vulgaris	St John's Wort	Hypericum perforatum
Celery	Apium graveolens	Lavender	Lavendula officinalis	Sweet flag	Acorus calamus
Chickweed	Stellaria media	Lemon	Citrus limon	Tea	Camellia sinensis
Chillies	Capsicum minimum	Lemon balm	Melissa officinalis	Thyme	Thymus vulgaris
Chinese rhubarb	Rheum palmatum	Lime	Tilia europea	Turmeric	Curcuma longa
Cinnamon	Cinnamonum verum	Liquorice	Glycyrrhiza glabra	Valerian	Valeriana officinalis
Cleavers	Galium aparine	Lovage	Levisticum officinale	Vervain	Verbena officinalis
Coltsfoot	Tussilago farfara	Marigold	Calendula officinalis	Wild cabbage	Brassica oleracea
Comfrey	Symphytum officinale	Marshmallow	Althea officinalis	Wild carrot	Daucus carota
Cornsilk	Zea mays	Meadowsweet	Filipendula ulmaria	Wild yam	Dioscorea villosa
Cramp bark	Viburnum opulus	Motherwort	Leonurus cardiaca	Willow	Salix alba
Dandelion	Taraxacum officinale	Mugwort	Artemisia vulgaris	Wormwood	Artemisia absinthium
Echinacea	Echinacea angustifolia	Mullein	Verbascum thapsus	Yarrow	Achillea millefolium
Elder	Sambucus nigra	Nettle	Urtica dioica		
Elecampane	Inula helenium	Oats	Avena sativa		

Achillea millefolium YARROW

Yarrow is a member of the daisy family which is native to Europe. It is widely distributed around pastureland, meadows, hedgerows and grassy verges, except in Mediterranean regions. It has now also colonised many of the English-speaking areas of the world, such as the United States, New Zealand and Australia. Yarrow has finely divided leaves (*millefolium* means 'a thousand leaves') and flat heads of tiny white, occasionally pink, flowers seen from June to September, when the herb is harvested. Since antiquity it has been a major herb in folk medicine throughout Europe. To gardeners, however, it is a troublesome weed, hard to eradicate because of its underground propagation. Yarrow's many active constituents include a light blue volatile oil (similar in many respects to camomile oil), tannins, alkaloids and a bitter principle.

Actions Yarrow has many traditional uses, yet it has never received extensive pharmacological investigation. Existing research, however, demonstrates its ability to reduce haemorrhaging, for example, and knowledge of many of its individual constituents supports most traditional uses. Among its country names, nosebleed, soldier's woundwort and staunchwort highlight yarrow's styptic, anti-inflammatory and antibacterial properties. It is also antispasmodic, hypotensive and diaphoretic, and can aid peripheral blood flow and warm the extremities – the hands and feet. These properties account for yarrow's long use as a tonic herb for circulatory problems of almost all kinds, from insufficiency to hypertension.

The volatile oil is responsible for several of yarrow's actions, being antispasmodic, carminative, anti-inflammatory and anthelminthic. Astringent and bitter properties added to its carminative actions make it an excellent digestive tonic. Like many antispasmodic herbs, yarrow is a uterine stimulant.

Uses As a circulatory herb, yarrow can aid hypertension, poor circulation and varicose veins. It also has applications in a wide range of digestive problems, including poor appetite, sluggish digestion, wind and belching, inflammation of the digestive system (which should receive professional treatment) and bowel irritability. Infusions of yarrow are helpful in relieving colds and chills and recovery from infections. Taken regularly in small doses yarrow helps to reduce excessive menstrual bleeding and cramps, and to regulate the menstrual cycle.

Dosage and preparations
Tincture – 1:5, 25%, 2–4 ml.
Infusion – 4 g per cup.

Cautions and contraindications
Avoid during pregnancy. A rare allergy to yarrow and some other herbs such as camomile, marigold and arnica causes temporary red pimply rashes. No other problems are known in normal use.

Achillea millefolium

Acorus calamus SWEET FLAG

A vigorous marsh-loving plant with sword-shaped leaves, sweet flag is native to temperate and sub-tropical regions. Introduced into the UK in the 1590s by the famous herbalist and gardener, John Gerard, it soon became a favourite herb for strewing over floors. Apart from its highly aromatic roots, the main active constituents are a volatile oil, a bitter principle and tannins.

Actions Sweet flag stimulates the production of saliva and is a stomach tonic, increasing secretions and stimulating the appetite. Mildly sedative, it is traditionally used in Asia as a nerve tonic.

Uses An excellent digestive herb, sweet flag is effective in easing heartburn, a poor appetite, poor digestion and the feeling of bloatedness after meals. It relaxes the bowel and eases colic and flatulence. These actions, coupled with sweet flag's mild sedative effect, make it useful in treating irritable bowel syndrome. The essential oil is very refreshing, especially for tired feet.

Dosage and preparations
Tincture – 1:5, 45%, 0.3–1 ml.
Infusion – 1 g per cup.

Cautions and contraindications
Large doses may irritate the digestive tract. Plants cultivated for essential oil are high in b-asarone, which is carcinogenic, so the essential oil should not be used internally. However, Indian mill workers chew the root regularly and there is no record of their suffering malignancy as a result.

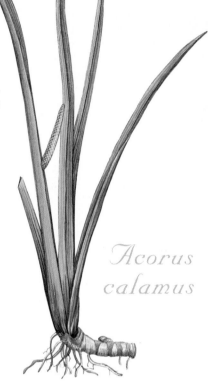

Acorus calamus

Aesculus hippocastanum HORSE CHESTNUT

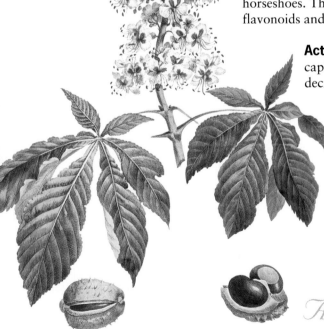

The horse chestnut is a native of northern and central Asia, introduced into England in the mid-1500s. This large, noble tree bears spikes of red-tinged, creamy-white flowers and has leaf scars on its branches in the exact shape of horseshoes. The seeds, familiarly known as conkers, contain saponins, flavonoids and tannins.

Actions Horse chestnut is an astringent tonic for the veins and capillaries, strengthening these vessels, improving blood flow and decreasing swelling. It is mildly anti-inflammatory and diuretic.

Uses Horse chestnut is a first-rate remedy, taken internally and used externally as an ointment for conditions where the veins are not functioning correctly, such as varicose veins and haemorrhoids.

Dosage and preparations
Tincture – 1:5, 25%, 0.5–2 ml.
Infusion – up to 1 g of crushed seeds in a cup with honey or other sweetener to mask the bitterness.
Ointment – add leaf juice or tincture to water soluble base.

Cautions and contraindications
People who suffer kidney disease or damage should avoid horse chestnut. If you are taking anticoagulant therapy (such as warfarin or aspirin), do not take horse chestnut except under professional supervision as it may strengthen the effects of your conventional medication.

Aesculus hippocastanum

Agrimonia eupatoria AGRIMONY

A pretty, straight-stemmed hedgerow plant, agrimony should be gathered from June, when the flowering yellow spikes appear, until the flowers die away. Agrimony contains a moderate quantity of tannins, which are drying and astringent, a little volatile oil and a bitter principle.

Actions Agrimony combines bitter digestive tonic effects with a mildly astringent action, toning and healing the mucous membranes of the gut. It helps to regulate the function of the liver and gallbladder and it has been used in Germany to treat gallstones and cirrhosis. Historically agrimony was greatly valued in wound-healing preparation and was used with mugwort and vinegar in the 'egrimoyne' of Chaucer's time. It was an ingredient in arquebusade water – named after harquebus, an early type of gun – used to treat gunshot wounds in Europe in the 16th century. Chinese research has proved its efficacy as a blood clotting agent.

Uses Helpful for treating diarrhoea or mild gastrointestinal infections, especially in children. Agrimony is also one of the herbs of choice for an irritable bowel and colicky pains, especially if often accompanied by loose motions. An infusion is effective and soothing as a gargle for sore throats or a mouthwash for sore gums and mouth ulcers.

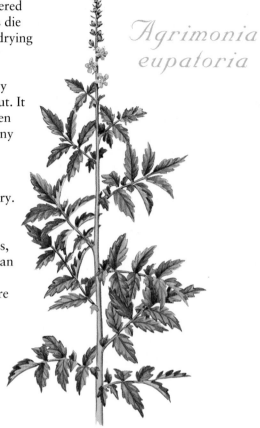

Agrimonia eupatoria

Dosage and preparations
Tincture – 1:5, 25%, 1–4 ml.
Infusion – 1–4 g steeped for 10 minutes.

Cautions and contraindications
None known.

Alchemilla vulgaris LADY'S MANTLE

Lady's mantle grows in pastures and hedgerows across northern Europe and Asia and over most of the UK and eastern USA, where it is widely cultivated in private gardens for its soft, pretty foliage. It has an unusual reproductive cycle – the seed develops without fertilisation from a male plant, a process known as parthenogenesis. The leaves and stems, which are collected between July and August, contain tannins and saponins.

Actions Lady's mantle has astringent and stomachic properties. It is often used as a digestive tonic, menstrual regulator and has a styptic action.

Uses Lady's mantle is a valuable herb for treating ailments of the female reproductive tract. It can be taken internally for irregular or excessive menstrual bleeding, for both of which professional advice should be sought, and for all menopausal symptoms. For external inflammation and itching an infusion of the fresh leaves can be applied topically to the affected area. A strong infusion taken frequently is a good treatment for mild diarrhoea, especially in children; it can also help to heal cuts and bruises when applied topically. For external applications, use either an infusion of the leaves or a decoction of the fresh root.

Alchemilla vulgaris

Dosage and preparations
Tincture – 1:5, 25%, or fresh, 1:2, 25%, 2–4 ml.
Infusion – 2 teaspoons per cup, infused for 10 minutes.

Cautions and contraindications
Not to be taken during pregnancy due to its styptic action.

Allium sativum GARLIC

Garlic cloves or corms (underground shoots) have been used medicinally, as well as in the kitchen, throughout known history. Grown all over the world, they contain a highly pungent volatile oil, minerals and abundant vitamins.

Actions Raw garlic is powerfully antibacterial and antifungal, especially one to three hours after crushing or bruising. Huge quantities of garlic were used during the First World War to disinfect wounds and prevent gangrene, just as they were by the Roman army over 2000 years earlier, and it has often been used as a precaution during infectious epidemics. Raw garlic is also effective against intestinal parasites and helps to strengthen and protect the digestive tract. Garlic's antiseptic, volatile substances are excreted through, and disinfect, the lungs, skin and urine, and thus the pungent odour is to some extent unavoidable.

Garlic has remarkable and well-researched positive effects on the heart and blood vessels, lowering blood pressure and cholesterol levels. It also adjusts the balance of fats in the blood, favouring those that inhibit furring of the arteries (atherosclerosis). Garlic can help to reduce the formation of clots in the blood vessels and help to break up those that have formed. In other words, it can be used to help reduce all of the major factors involved in degenerative heart disease.

Uses Garlic is used in the treatment of viral, bacterial and fungal infections, whether internal or external, and has been proven very useful for relieving gastrointestinal infections. When applied externally it can help to combat fungal infections such as vaginal thrush and athlete's foot, and help to clean infected wounds. Internally it is highly effective for keeping colds at bay. Garlic should be taken daily by anyone with a personal or family history of raised cholesterol, high blood pressure or heart problems. Regular garlic intake is also beneficial for sluggish digestion, with wind and bloating, especially in older people.

Allium sativum

Dosage and preparations

For infection, infestation of the digestive tract, and prevention of colds and 'flu, take one raw clove per day that has been bruised, chopped, or infused and left to cool. In acute infections, this quantity can be doubled. For problems of the circulation, take at least half a clove per day, dried, fresh, or in tablets, capsules or perls. For external application use a garlic infusion in a compress or cream.

Cautions and contraindications

Although generally very safe, garlic can irritate a sensitive digestion. Lowering the dose and taking infusions may help. To help reduce 'garlic breath', chew a sprig of parsley or eat an apple after taking garlic. Do not use raw garlic directly on the skin – it can cause burns.

Allium cepa ONION

Onions have been cultivated for over 6000 years and their medicinal benefits have come to be widely applauded. They share many of the constituents of garlic, including vitamin C, minerals, flavonoids and a volatile oil.

Actions As with garlic (see page 89), the expectorant, antibacterial and antifungal properties of onion are most effective after crushing or bruising. Onions have a beneficial action on lipids in the blood, reducing the effects of dietary saturated fats and the build up of fatty plaques. They also counteract rises in blood sugar, reduce blood clotting and are believed to significantly reduce the risk of some cancers, especially that of the stomach.

Uses Onion is a very versatile household medicine. A small piece, lightly boiled, placed in the outer part of the ear can help to relieve the pain of earache, and fresh syrup of onion is an excellent disinfecting expectorant. A compress of roasted onion placed on the painful joint may help to relieve the discomfort of gout.

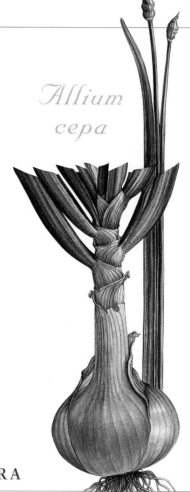

Allium cepa

Dosage and preparations
To achieve beneficial changes in blood lipids and the anti-infective effects you need to eat at least half a strong, raw onion every day. For other effects, cooked onions will suffice. A syrup can be made by putting equal amounts of sliced onion and sugar in a jar and draining off the resulting fluid a few hours later.

Cautions and contraindications
Raw onions may be overheating or excessively stimulating to some people, causing indigestion.

Aloe vera ALOE VERA

Aloe vera

A large succulent tropical plant, which can easily be grown as a houseplant, aloe vera has a ring of spiny, fleshy white-flecked leaves. The laxative juice from these leaves has long been used medicinally and is usually dried and sold as resin. The gel, exuded naturally when a leaf tip is cut, has antibiotic principles and has become very popular following its use as a healing agent in the Second World War.

Actions The bitter juice or resin is irritating to the bowel and has a cathartic action. The gel is a powerful healing agent, encouraging skin regeneration, yet is gentle enough to use directly on burns and wounds. It is also bacteriocidal and mildly laxative.

Uses Aloe vera gel is healing for mouth and skin ulcers, burns, wounds and dry skin, sunburn and radiation burns. It also has a reputation, which is not yet adequately researched, for relieving gastrointestinal inflammation and calming an irritable bowel.

Dosage and preparations
Use the fresh gel or preparations rich in it, as required. There are high and low quality preparations available to buy in health food shops and chemists.

Cautions and contraindications
Aloe resin is not recommended for home use, but it may be a component of proprietary laxatives. Do not take these for more than a week as they may lead to bowel flaccidity and mineral loss. Aloe gel seems to be very safe for both external and internal use.

Alpinia officinarum GALANGAL

Galangal is a medium to tall east Asian herb belonging to the same family as ginger. It has reed-like leaves and a cluster of white flowers. The rhizomes (root branches) have been used medicinally in Europe for over 1000 years and are known to have been used by Arabs to make their horses more 'fiery'. The rhizomes smell pungent and spicy and have a taste similar to ginger. Galangal root contains volatile oil and resin.

Actions Galangal has similar properties to ginger, but is gentler and less pungent. It is a diaphoretic, a circulatory stimulant, an aromatic digestive tonic and a carminative.

Uses Galangal is mainly used for digestive complaints, particularly flatulence and sluggish digestion which causes, for example, bloating, colic and wind after large meals. Like ginger, it can be used to prevent travel sickness and to quell other feelings of nausea. Its warming, diaphoretic effects make it a useful herb for fevers, though less stimulating than cinnamon, cayenne or ginger.

Dosage and preparations
Tincture – 1:5, 45%, 0.5–2 ml.
Infusion – 1–3 ml if powdered.
Decoction – 1 g per cup.

Cautions and contraindications
None known.

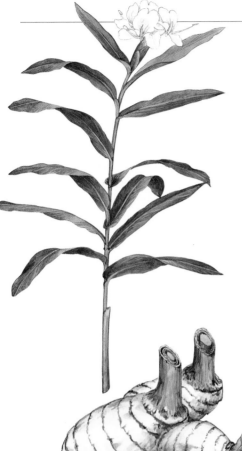

Alpinia officinarum

Althea officinalis MARSHMALLOW

Marshmallow is a perennial, seashore-loving plant that grows in temperate regions worldwide. Its pink flowers grow on tall stems which are covered, like the leaves, with soft, velvety down. The leaves, and especially the roots, contain mucilage whilst the leaves and flowers contain a little volatile oil.

Actions The mucilage contained within the leaves and roots is a complex starch which absorbs water and becomes demulcent and emollient. The flowers and leaves are a soothing expectorant.

Uses Marshmallow leaves and flowers are useful for dry, congested coughs and for cystitis. If boiled in distilled water the leaves are also soothing for conjunctivitis. The infusion makes an excellent gargle and mouthwash for hoarseness, oral thrush and gum abscesses. The root is primarily used for acid indigestion and diarrhoea, although it also gives softness and bulk to stools and so may help to relieve constipation. When given to teething babies to chew, chunks of the peeled root are excellent for soothing the gums, and the dried root powder is a good drawing compound for splinters and boils.

Dosage and preparations
Tincture – 1:5, 25%, 2–4 ml.
Infusion – root: 1 part herb to 20 parts water, soak for 1–2 hours, then gently heat to 50°C (122°F) and leave to cool. Leaf/flower: 2 g per cup infused for 10 minutes.

Cautions and contraindications
None known.

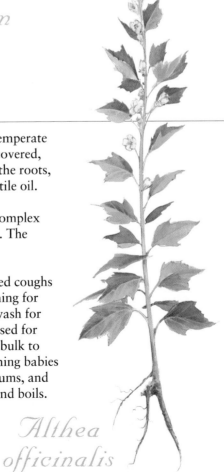

Althea officinalis

Angelica archangelica ANGELICA

Angelica is an impressive plant which grows up to 2 m (6 ft 6 in) tall and is as widely cultivated for its appearance as for its candied stems used in baking. The root, containing volatile oil, resin and a bitter principle, is harvested at the end of the plant's first year in autumn or early spring. The leaves, which are also used occasionally, should be collected in June.

Actions Angelica is a warming, circulatory stimulant as well as being expectorant and antispasmodic. It is an excellent digestive tonic and is very useful in relieving loss of appetite and debility. It also has a long history of use as a general restorative.

Uses Angelica is one of the most widely used aromatic remedies and is helpful in convalescence, for poor circulation and for coughs. An infused oil of angelica and fennel is a good warming rub for a tight chest and the candied flower stalks, used in cake decoration, are also therapeutic for children with weak chests. The leaf has a more gentle action than the root and is therefore more suited to treating children's complaints.

Dosage and preparations
Tincture – 1:5, 45%, 0.5–2 ml.

Cautions and contraindications
Some people are sensitive to angelica and can develop a rash from handling the plant in sunlight.

Angelica archangelica

Apium graveolens CELERY

A popular salad vegetable, especially with slimmers because of its very low calorie and high fibre content, celery is native to southern Europe, but widely cultivated in Britain. Its name, *graveolens* means 'strong smelling'. The seeds, the main medicinal part of the herb, are used as a condiment and a salt substitute. They contain a volatile oil, coumarins and flavonoids.

Actions Celery seeds have a mild diuretic and cleansing action and are believed to assist the elimination of uric acid, a build-up of which can lead to gout and kidney stones. They also have mild sedative properties.

Uses Celery seeds work particularly well alongside diuretics like dandelion leaf, and can be helpful in the treatment of arthritis and gout. They are also helpful in settling a sensitive digestion as they are mildly antispasmodic. The root, and to a lesser extent the stalks, share the actions of the seeds, and arthritis sufferers are recommended to eat plenty of celery.

Dosage and preparations
Tincture – 1:3, 45%, 2–5 ml.
Infusion – 5 g per cup, or added to dandelion leaf infusion.

Cautions and contraindications
People suffering from kidney inflammation should avoid celery seed.

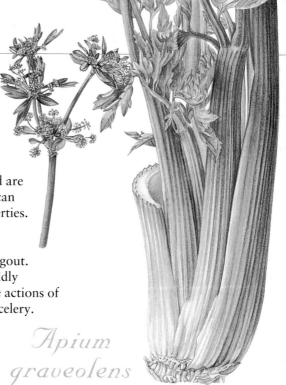

Apium graveolens

92

Arctium lappa BURDOCK

A magnificent plant with large, soft, heart-shaped leaves and round heads of purple flowers, burdock grows on wasteland and in hedgerows. The seed heads, covered with hooked spines which stick to fur and clothing, have attracted names such as 'beggar's buttons' and 'thorny burr'. The sweet, mucilaginous root grows up to 1 m (3 ft) long and is harvested in the plant's first year. The burdock root contains a trace of volatile oil and the seeds and leaves are also used medicinally.

Actions With its hypoglycaemic, diaphoretic and mildly diuretic actions, burdock appears to help to move toxins from the tissues into the bloodstream to be removed by the kidneys and to some extent the skin and lungs. Burdock also has a bacteriostatic action.

Uses Burdock's main use is for skin problems such as acne, eczema and psoriasis, and for arthritis and other congestion-related conditions. It should be taken over long periods of time, in small doses at first. The leaf and root are both used externally in soothing topical applications.

Arctium lappa

Dosage and preparations
Tincture – 1:5, 25%, 2–8 ml.
Decoction – 3 g per cup.
The fresh leaf juice, from health food shops or home-made, can be refrigerated or frozen.

Cautions and contraindications
Avoid large doses at first to avoid overloading channels of toxin elimination, such as skin pores and kidneys.

Artemisia absinthium WORMWOOD
Artemisia vulgaris MUGWORT

Wormwood has grey-green hairy stems and feathery leaves. Mugwort produces clusters of small red or yellow flowers and dark green, deeply indented leaves. Both can grow to 1 m (3 ft) tall. Mugwort is more common on the roadsides of the UK while wormwood is found in coastal areas, but both grow widely in temperate regions and help to deter midges. Most medieval herbals refer to mugwort as motherwort (for the womb). Both contain bitter glycosides, volatile oil and tannins.

Actions Mugwort is a digestive tonic with a warming, aromatic, bitter action and a slightly stimulating nervous restorative. It also eases uterine problems. Wormwood is a more bitter and powerful digestive stimulant which is anthelminthic.

Uses Mugwort helps to regulate irregular periods, aids digestive debility associated with fatigue and is traditionally taken for strengthening eyesight. Wormwood is used for poor digestion, the inability to digest fats and loss of appetite associated with depression or convalescence. It also fights worm infestations.

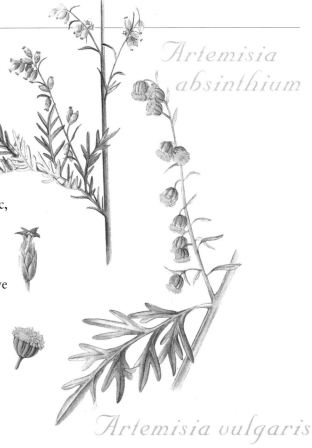

Artemisia absinthium

Artemisia vulgaris

Dosage and preparations
Tinctures – both 1:5, 25%, 0.5–2 ml.
Infusions – mugwort 1–4 g, wormwood 1–2 g.
Wormwood can be used in the form of pills or capsules for worm infestations, but do not use more than 2 g, three times a day.

Cautions and contraindications
Avoid during pregnancy.
Both herbs need to be taken very cautiously because large amounts can cause nerve damage.

Avena sativa OATS

Oats grow wild in temperate and cool climates and are widely cultivated all over the world as a food crop. The whole plant is used medicinally and is harvested when the seeds are developing in midsummer. Active ingredients include alkaloids, saponins, minerals and B vitamins.

Actions Oatstraw is a major nervous restorative which nourishes, sustains and calms the nervous system whilst enhancing mood. Oat grains are very high in soluble fibre, which can help to soothe the digestive tract, improve bowel motility ('keeping you regular') and lower cholesterol levels.

Uses Oats are good for convalescence or for nervous debility, especially after conditions such as neuralgia and shingles. A useful alternative to oatstraw preparations is oatmeal soaked overnight in water. This can also make a soothing application for dry and irritable skin.

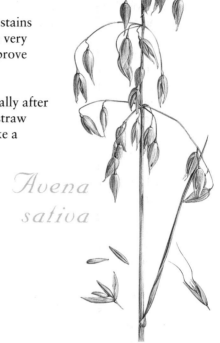

Avena sativa

Dosage and preparations
Tincture – (oatstraw) 1:3, 25%, 1–2 ml doses when needed. Decoction – 20 g to 600 ml. Alternatively, 20 g oatmeal soaked overnight and taken in the morning.

Cautions and contraindications
Taken in large doses, oats can cause headaches. Oatmeal and porridge contain gluten, so gluten-sensitive people should avoid them, although the tincture and decoction should be gluten-free if left to settle and separated from the sediment.

Borago officinalis BORAGE

A rough hairy perennial, borage has blue, star-shaped flowers which attract bees and provide delicious honey. It is naturalised across Europe and common in the UK in kitchen gardens and near dwellings. The seeds contain g-linoleic acid, a plant acid essential in nutrition, even more than is found in evening primrose seeds.

Actions The leaves and flowers of borage are diaphoretic, restorative, demulcent, galactogogue and emollient. Dioscorides, a Roman army physician and author of the famous herbal *Materia Medica*, wrote that borage 'cheers the heart and raises the spirits'. Herbalists today use it to alleviate symptoms of stress and as a nerve restorative, an antidepressant and to help support the adrenal production of hormones that regulate the body's systems.

Uses Traditionally, borage has been used to treat inflammation of the digestive tract, but has also found a place in the treatment of depression and nervous exhaustion. The hot infusion induces sweating in fevers, while the flowers can be used to flavour summer wine (giving a cucumber-like taste) and the young leaves add flavour to salads.

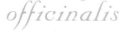

Borago officinalis

Dosage and preparations
Tincture – 1:5, 25%, 1–2 ml.
Infusion – 2 g per cup.
Summer wine cup – borage, lemon, sugar, wine, water, mixed to taste and chilled. Borage is best used fresh.

Cautions and contraindications
Borage contains alkaloids which, when taken in isolation, can cause liver damage. It is therefore not recommended for prolonged internal use.

94

Calendula officinalis MARIGOLD

Marigold is a yellow or bright orange garden annual which likes sunny positions. It is native to the same regions as the vine and can be found in vineyards, cultivated fields and gardens. Double flowers, from modern orange hybrids, are preferred medicinally, as the ray florets – parts of the flowerhead which look like petals but are in reality each a tiny flower – contain the major medicinally valuable constituents.

Actions Marigold flowers are decongestant, astringent and help to heal tissue when applied topically. They have anti-inflammatory properties and are mildly diaphoretic and stimulating to the circulation. They are also, mainly through their gum and resin content, antifungal, antibacterial and antiprotozoal – protozoa are single cell organisms, one type of which is responsible for malaria – but because these principles are not water soluble, preserving them requires a tincture very high in ethanol or an oil. A water-based extract has anti-inflammatory and antiviral properties whilst also helping to boost the immune system.

Uses Marigold is an excellent treatment for chronic infections and chronic skin disorders, whether taken orally or applied externally. It is particularly useful (under professional guidance) in treating gastric infections and ulcers. The infusion helps to bring on delayed periods and alleviate menstrual pain.

A compress or a poultice using marigold is an excellent first aid treatment for burns, scalds, stings and impetigo – a highly contagious skin disorder – helping to soothe and heal. A cream or compress is also helpful for varicose veins, chilblains and broken skin. A mouthwash or gargle is useful for mouth ulcers, gum disease and throat infections.

An ointment or cream containing the tincture or infused oil, especially in combination with myrrh tincture or essential oil and tea tree essential oil, is an effective local treatment for fungal infections affecting the skin, nails, feet (athlete's foot, for example), or the vaginal area (such as thrush). A lotion made from an infusion also makes a useful compress for sore or inflamed eyes.

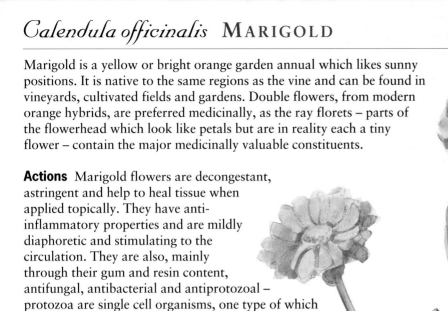

Calendula officinalis

Dosages and preparations
Tincture – 1:5, 25%, 0.5–2 ml.
Tincture to extract antibacterial gums and resins –
1:5, 90%, 0.5–1.5 ml.
Infusion – 1–2 g infused for 5–10 minutes.
Infused oil – heat gently in sunflower oil.
A cream combining all of the therapeutic actions
may be made by combining the water-based
extract with oil or strong alcohol-based extracts.

Cautions and contraindications
Avoid during pregnancy because of its
emmenagogue action.

Brassica oleracea WILD CABBAGE

Relatives of the cabbage include herbs such as hedge garlic, black mustard, horseradish, shepherd's purse and vegetables of the brassica family. Most share common constituents known as isothiocyanates, or mustard oil, the acrid, irritating basis of the mustard gas used in the First World War. Nonetheless, cabbage is medicinally useful in its natural state.

Actions Cabbage has two well-researched properties. First, cabbage-leaf juice has been found to be beneficial in healing peptic ulcers. Second, cabbage in any form is believed to play a role in the prevention of cancers, particularly colo-rectal cancers. It is thought that the cabbage's antimutagenic effect that opposes and suppresses mutation or abnormal changes in the cells derives from a natural defence against irritants. The bruised leaves, applied to the skin, have anti-inflammatory, anti-infective and circulatory stimulant effects.

Uses The juice, taken in small, frequent doses over several weeks alongside other medications, is recommended for duodenal ulcers. A diet rich in cabbage and the other members of the brassica family, such as brussels sprouts and broccoli, is recommended for people with a family history of bowel cancer. Applications of the bruised leaf are useful for both mastitis and hot, painful arthritic joints.

Brassica oleracea

Dosage and preparations
Fresh cabbage juice – 20–50 ml taken every few hours. Other preparations as above.

Cautions and contraindications
None known.

Camellia sinensis TEA

Tea is a perennial evergreen that grows in tropical or sub-tropical areas. Archaeological evidence shows that tea was known 500 000 years ago, and as a beverage it is now second only to water in worldwide popularity. For black tea, commonly drunk in the West, the leaves are allowed to ferment after picking, whereas green tea, popular in the East, is brewed using unfermented leaves. Infusions contain polyphenols (tannin-like substances) and caffeine.

Actions Tea's paradoxical stimulating and calming effects on the nervous system are well known, but are pharmacologically complex. Evidence from studies suggests a protective effect, especially from green tea, against cancers of the digestive tract, particularly the mouth, oesophagus, stomach, pancreas and colon. This may be due partly to its inactivation of carcinogens in cooked meat and fish and partly to its antioxidant effects. Drinking tea may also help to prevent strokes and fatty deposits in the arteries.

Uses Green tea drunk without milk may help to prevent cardiovascular problems and reduce the risk of some cancers. Black tea without milk is a good treatment for, as well as preventing attacks of, diarrhoea.

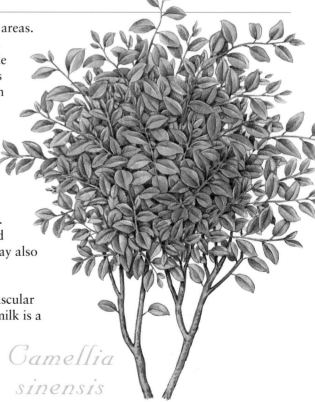

Camellia sinensis

Dosage and preparations
Tea can be drunk as an infusion, made to taste.

Cautions and contraindications
Large quantities of tea, especially taken without milk, may decrease absorption of nutrients, especially iron.

Chamomilla recutita CAMOMILE

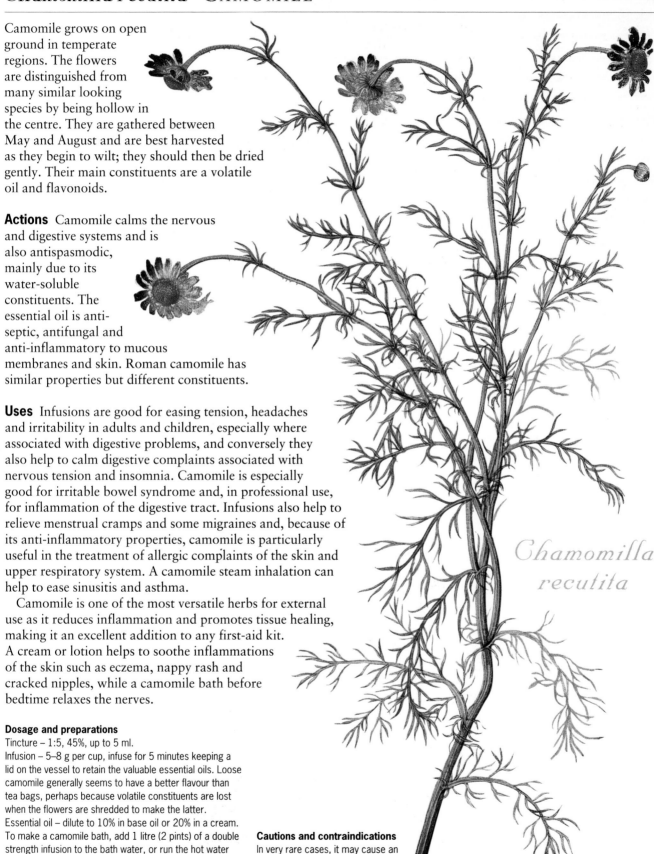

Camomile grows on open ground in temperate regions. The flowers are distinguished from many similar looking species by being hollow in the centre. They are gathered between May and August and are best harvested as they begin to wilt; they should then be dried gently. Their main constituents are a volatile oil and flavonoids.

Actions Camomile calms the nervous and digestive systems and is also antispasmodic, mainly due to its water-soluble constituents. The essential oil is anti-septic, antifungal and anti-inflammatory to mucous membranes and skin. Roman camomile has similar properties but different constituents.

Uses Infusions are good for easing tension, headaches and irritability in adults and children, especially where associated with digestive problems, and conversely they also help to calm digestive complaints associated with nervous tension and insomnia. Camomile is especially good for irritable bowel syndrome and, in professional use, for inflammation of the digestive tract. Infusions also help to relieve menstrual cramps and some migraines and, because of its anti-inflammatory properties, camomile is particularly useful in the treatment of allergic complaints of the skin and upper respiratory system. A camomile steam inhalation can help to ease sinusitis and asthma.

Camomile is one of the most versatile herbs for external use as it reduces inflammation and promotes tissue healing, making it an excellent addition to any first-aid kit. A cream or lotion helps to soothe inflammations of the skin such as eczema, nappy rash and cracked nipples, while a camomile bath before bedtime relaxes the nerves.

Chamomilla recutita

Dosage and preparations
Tincture – 1:5, 45%, up to 5 ml.
Infusion – 5–8 g per cup, infuse for 5 minutes keeping a lid on the vessel to retain the valuable essential oils. Loose camomile generally seems to have a better flavour than tea bags, perhaps because volatile constituents are lost when the flowers are shredded to make the latter.
Essential oil – dilute to 10% in base oil or 20% in a cream. To make a camomile bath, add 1 litre (2 pints) of a double strength infusion to the bath water, or run the hot water through a muslin or cloth bag filled with camomile flowers, as you fill the bath.

Cautions and contraindications
In very rare cases, it may cause an allergic rash. Discontinue oral or topical treatment in this case.

Capsella bursa-pastoris SHEPHERD'S PURSE

Probably of European or western Asian origin, but now found worldwide with the exception of the tropics, shepherd's purse is one of the most common weeds. They can grow from a single small stem in a pavement crack to a bush on wasteland. The name refers to the plant's distinctive flat seed-pods. Shepherd's purse contains flavonoids and saponins.

Actions Shepherd's purse is styptic, astringent and a urinary antiseptic. Its styptic action, confirmed by research, is mild, but its leaves were used to staunch bleeding during the First World War in the absence of ergot, a styptic fungus that grows on cereals which was used to treat wounds in the trenches. Shepherd's purse also causes the uterus to contract and is a mild circulatory stimulant.

Uses Traditionally, shepherd's purse was used for all forms of internal bleeding. It is now, however, used specifically for heavy menstrual bleeding and it should be combined with other herbs that address any hormonal cause of this problem. It can also be used to treat diarrhoea and cystitis.

Capsella bursa-pastoris

Dosage and preparations
Tincture – 1:5, 25%, 1–5 ml.
Infusion – 5 g per cup, steeped
for 10 minutes.

Cautions and contraindications
Shepherd's purse should not be taken
in pregnancy, but otherwise is safe.

Capsicum minimum CHILLIES

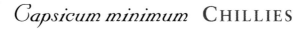

Chillies are a variety of capsicum, a small upright tropical shrub, closely related to red and green peppers, tomatoes, potatoes, tobacco and deadly nightshade. The name *capsicum* derives from an ancient Greek word for 'box'. The fiery-tasting alkaloid, capsaicin, gives chillies their distinctive 'heat' and they also contain beta-carotene and vitamin C.

Actions A general stimulant, cayenne (chilli pepper) is also a digestive and circulatory tonic, an anticoagulant, an antispasmodic and an analgesic. It is expectorant and decongestant and thins secretions, such as phlegm and mucus. Cayenne's remarkable range of actions are associated with its powerful heating and stimulating properties.

Uses Cayenne stimulates the appetite and is particularly useful for sluggish digestion, especially in the elderly, and for colic and flatulence. It is a heating circulatory stimulant, useful to stave off the start of a cold or chill. Used externally it produces redness and warmth, relieving stiff joints and nerve or muscle pain. It loosens catarrh and mucus in bronchitis.

Capsicum minimum

Dosage and preparations
Tincture – 1:10, 60%, 0.3–1ml,
well diluted.
Powder – 30–50 mg.
The powder can be infused in oil
or added to a cream for external
application.

Cautions and contraindications
Use in small quantities. Not
recommended for sufferers of
hypertension or gastric irritation except
under professional supervision. Can
occasionally produce a pustular rash
on the skin.

Cinnamonum verum CINNAMON

Cinnamon is the inner bark from a tropical tree, native to Sri Lanka, which can grow to 10 m (35 ft) high. Types of cinnamon include Ceylon cinnamon (*Cinnamonum zeylanicum*) which is more fragrant than Chinese cinnamon (*Cinnamonum cassia*), called cassia. Ceylon cinnamon is also more commonly available in the UK. The main constituents are a volatile oil, coumarins and tannins.

Actions Cinnamon is a warming digestive stimulant and also a circulatory stimulant. It is antispasmodic and a carminative with an antidiarrhoeal effect and acts to improve the action of the stomach and digestive secretions.

Uses Cinnamon is very effective for poor appetite, especially associated with sluggish digestion and a feeling of coldness. The warming effect is useful in treating chesty colds, especially when mixed with ginger, or influenza when mixed with elderflower and peppermint. It is an important spice in mulled wine, as it helps to keep out the winter cold. Taking a cinnamon infusion helps sufferers of cold hands and feet, and is a useful general tonic in prolonged illness.

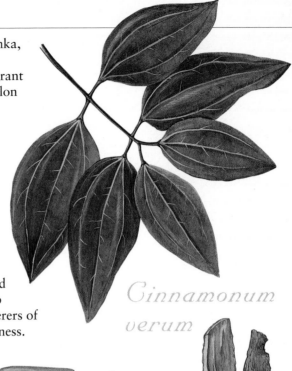

Cinnamonum verum

Dosage and preparations
Tincture – 1:5, 45%, 0.3–1 ml.
Infusion – 0.5–1 g, taken as necessary for colds and flu.

Cautions and contraindications
Do not take during pregnancy as it may cause miscarriage.

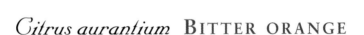

Citrus aurantium BITTER ORANGE

The Arabs were the first recorded people to have cultivated bitter oranges and they are now widely grown in all Mediterranean countries. They are rich in vitamin C and contain flavonoids in the peel.

Actions Consumption of any citrus fruit can help to protect against cancer of the stomach, oesophagus and possibly of the pancreas. The juice is effective against some viruses and the pectin in the skin and membranes of both oranges and grapefruit has been found to help lower blood cholesterol.

Uses Infusions of bitter orange peel and orange flowers are good for insomnia. Dried bitter orange peel was used as a digestive tonic in the West and is used as a warming stomachic in Chinese medicine. Bitter orange flowers yield a fragrant and expensive volatile oil – neroli – which is used in high-quality perfumes and aromatherapy. An infusion of the flowers is also useful.

Citrus aurantium

Dosage and preparations
For the full cardiovascular benefits of oranges, eat the pithy parts and the membranes as well as the flesh and add the zest to orange juice. The vitamin C is quickly lost to the air so drink the juice straight after pouring.
Infusion – (orange flower or peel) 2–3 g per cup, steeped for 5 minutes.

Cautions and contraindications
This fruit may sometimes aggravate inflammatory conditions and hyperactivity in children.

Citrus limon LEMON

Citrus limon

Renowned through the ages as a health-giving fruit, lemons are very rich in vitamin C. One of the most famous medicinal uses of citrus fruit came about through an old British Navy regulation that stipulated an ounce of lemon or lime juice a day for every sailor after ten days at sea to prevent scurvy – hence the nickname 'limeys'.

Actions Lemon juice is disinfecting, antiviral, expectorant and astringent. The peel and pith are high in bioflavonoids, and are thought to be anticarcinogenic and able, in large amounts, to lower blood cholesterol. Lemon yields a refreshing volatile oil.

Uses The juice with water is an excellent gargle for sore throats. Honey and lemon infusions are disinfecting and mildly expectorant for colds and fevers. The oil is effective topically for viral warts such as verrucas. A Chinese remedy for whitlows (a strain of herpes found on the finger) is to bind the finger overnight inside a lemon.

Dosage and preparations
Infusion – 2 slices per cup for colds, combined with honey and ginger or cinnamon.
Essential oil – use directly on the wart but avoid contact with surrounding skin.
To gargle, dilute the juice of half a lemon in a wine glass of warm water.

Cautions and contraindications
The essential oil is irritating and lemon juice erodes tooth enamel, so rinse your teeth with water after contact. Lemon also has a reputation for leaching calcium, so take a supplement in moderation to compensate.

Cratageus oxyacantha HAWTHORN

Also known as mayflower, hawthorn's pink and white blossoms are a familiar sight in hedgerows throughout the UK in May and June, and are replaced by their red berries in September. The species hybridise freely and the leaves, flowering tops and berries all have similar properties. The leaves in particular are rich in glycosides and tannins.

Actions The properties of some of hawthorn's active constituents are well understood and present a remarkable picture of what herbalists refer to as synergy – meaning 'working together'. Some constituents strengthen the heart's action, others slow it slightly and improve its blood supply. The net effect is to make a weak heart work more efficiently and to reduce blood pressure. Hawthorn must be used long-term to have any significant effect.

Uses A good herb to take daily – alongside garlic – for anyone over 40 years old and with a history of hypertension or heart disease in the family. It is helpful for most degenerative conditions of the heart or blood vessels as a supplement to other therapies.

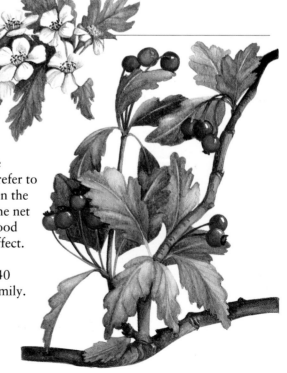

Cratageus oxyacantha

Dosage and preparations
Tincture – 1:5, 25%, 1–2 ml.
Infusion – 5 g of flowers and leaves per cup.

Cautions and contraindications
No known side effects, but if you are taking medicine for arrhythmias or heart failure, especially digoxin, use hawthorn only under professional supervision.

Curcuma longa TURMERIC

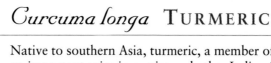

Native to southern Asia, turmeric, a member of the same family as ginger, is an important spice in curries and other Indian food. It contains a volatile oil, vitamins, minerals and the pigment curcumin, which is a common yellow-orange colouring agent in foods.

Actions The alkaloid curcumin in turmeric produces anticlotting, anti-inflammatory and antioxidant properties. Turmeric is also carminative, soothing to the digestion, and cholagogue, restorative to the liver.

Uses Turmeric is a valuable herb in treating gall bladder and liver problems and helpful in poor digestion associated with chronic fatigue and inflammation. It has proven anti-inflammatory effects that are very helpful in relieving the pain of rheumatoid arthritis. As an antioxidant, turmeric is recommended for degenerative circulatory disorders and it shares many uses with its relation, ginger, such as improving circulation, calming inflammation and detoxifying the body. It is used in China for shoulder pain and menstrual cramps and in India for liver disease.

Curcuma longa

Dosage and preparations
Powdered herb – 1–3 g per day, mixed into a thick liquid, such as apple or pear concentrate, or made into pills with honey.

Cautions and contraindications
None known. Care is needed when handling turmeric because it is liable to stain clothes, vessels and surfaces.

Daucus carota WILD CARROT

Wild carrot grows mainly in coastal regions in the UK. It is the same species as cultivated carrot, but the root is pale in colour, acrid to taste and very aromatic. Its leaves and seeds contain a volatile oil and an alkaloid; the roots of both varieties are rich in bioflavonoids, including beta-carotene, minerals and vitamins B_1, B_2 and C.

Actions The roots of both wild and cultivated carrots are soothing to the digestive system and seem to be powerfully protective against some cancers, notably those of the lung, colon and pancreas, probably due to the bioflavonoids. Wild carrot seeds and, to a lesser extent the aerial parts of the plant (leaves, stalk and flowers), are carminative, antiseptic and diuretic.

Uses Carrots are a valuable food, particularly suited to those with a sensitive digestion and, eaten 2 or 3 times a week, can help to improve night vision. Two or more carrots a day may give significant protection against many forms of cancer. Infusions or tinctures of the seeds, together with frequent drinks of water, ease flatulence, and are useful for treating cystitis or prostatitis. It also helps to flush out kidney stones.

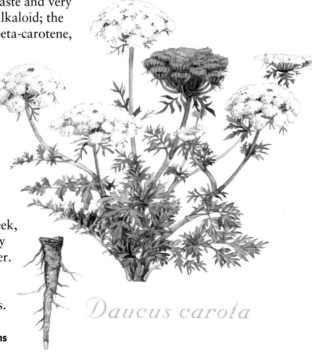

Daucus carota

Dosage and preparations
Tincture – (herb and seed) 1:5, 45%, 1–2 ml.
Infusion – (herb and seed) 1–2 g per cup steeped for 10 minutes.

Cautions and contraindications
Do not take carrot seeds during pregnancy.

Dioscorea villosa WILD YAM

Wild yam, as the name suggests, is the wild relative of the edible yam, a native of Mexico and the southern USA. It has a densely matted rootstock which contains steroidal saponins, alkaloids, tannins and starch.

Actions Wild yam is anti-inflammatory, antirheumatic and antispasmodic. It also has the effect of being diaphoretic and cholagogue. Its anti-inflammatory action may be due to the steroidal saponins. These have been used as a raw material for the production of the progesterone-only contraceptive pill and, although they are not converted in the body to progesterone, they are likely to have an influence on steroid hormone function.

Uses Wild yam is useful for inflammation and colicky conditions of the digestive tract, such as irritable bowel syndrome, stomach cramps and inflammatory bowel disease (only under professional guidance). It is also a major anti-inflammatory herb and is helpful in inflammatory conditions, such as rheumatoid arthritis. In recent years it has been seen more as a hormonal tonic and is useful for weakened hormonal production, menstrual pain and menopausal problems, particularly cramps and lack of energy.

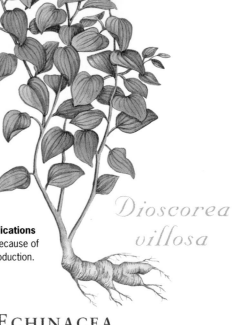

Dioscorea villosa

Dosage and preparations
Tincture – 1:5, 45%, 2–10 ml.
Decoction – 1 teaspoon per cup, simmered for 20 minutes.

Cautions and contraindications
Avoid during pregnancy because of the effect on hormone production.

Echinacea angustifolia ECHINACEA

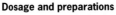

Echinacea is native to the USA, though purple coneflower (*Echinacea purpurea*) is now widely cultivated around the world. With distinctive large-petalled purple flowers, echinacea can reach up to 2 m (6 ft) in height. The root has a distinctive aroma and chewing it causes a numbness in the mouth. The root and rhizome, and occasionally aerial parts, are used and contain a volatile oil, glycosides, polysaccharides and a resin.

Actions Echinacea is a well-researched immune stimulant and a powerful tissue cleanser with vulnerary properties. It has antibacterial and antiviral properties and is particularly effective against herpes and influenza viruses. It is also mildly diaphoretic.

Uses Echinacea was a major medicine used by indigenous Americans for wounds, snake bites and fevers. It is excellent for ear, nose, throat and bronchial infections, especially those that are prolonged and accompanied by a cold. It has been found to be very useful in treating colds and flu because of its mild diaphoretic, immune system-stimulating and antiviral actions. As a tissue cleanser, echinacea can be used to treat boils and abscesses and can be applied externally to skin ulcers, infected wounds and vaginal infections, and taken as a gargle for throat infections.

Echinacea angustifolia

Dosage and preparations
Tincture – 1:5, 45%, 1–3 ml.
Infusion – 1–2 g per cup infused for 10 minutes.

Cautions and contraindications
None known. Can be taken in conjunction with antibiotics.

Equisetum arvense HORSETAIL

Horsetails are a primitive, non-flowering family of plants which reproduce by releasing spores. Their giant ancestors, along with ferns, once covered the planet and their fossils form our coal seams. Horsetail grows on wasteland, often above underground streams. The long green sterile stems make the best harvest and are gathered in summer, rather than the brownish fertile stems seen in spring. They contain flavonoids and minerals. Correct identification is crucial because horsetail's relative, mare's tail, contains a toxic alkaloid.

Actions With anti-inflammatory and astringent actions to the genito-urinary tract, horsetail is also mildly diuretic. It aids blood clotting and is used to heal connective tissue, particularly for damaged lungs and arthritic joints.

Uses Useful in treating mild cystitis and bed-wetting, horsetail has a long history of use for rheumatic conditions and may help to repair sprains, fractures and weak or brittle nails. Externally, a useful styptic and healing agent for wounds.

Dosage and preparations
Decoction – to draw out the active ingredients, grind and boil the herb for several hours. Use 25 g of horsetail per 600 ml of water, with a little sugar.

Cautions and contraindications
Inadvisable for people with heart or kidney disease, but otherwise safe.

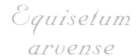

Equisetum arvense

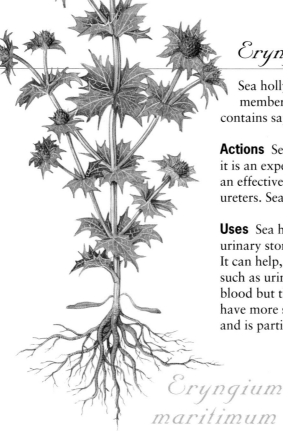

Eryngium maritimum SEA HOLLY

Sea holly is quite common on the sandy shores of northern Europe. It is a member of the carrot family but in appearance is more like a thistle. It contains saponins, flavonoids and the aromatic substance coumarin.

Actions Sea holly root shares many of the properties of angelica root in that it is an expectorant, a diaphoretic and a nervous system restorative. It is also an effective, relaxing diuretic, which increases urinary output and relaxes the ureters. Sea holly was once very popular candied, although this is now rare.

Uses Sea holly has traditionally been used to relieve renal colic and to clear urinary stones. It is also helpful for easing the pain of cystitis and prostatitis. It can help, especially in combination with horsetail, to relieve symptoms such as urinary frequency, irritation and the passing of small amounts of blood but these symptoms need professional evaluation because they can have more serious connotations. Sea holly can also be used to relieve coughs, and is particularly noted for whooping cough.

Dosage and preparations
Tincture – 1:5, 25%, 5–8 ml.
Infusion – 1 teaspoon of shredded root per cup, steep for 10 minutes.

Cautions and contraindications
The appearance of blood in the urine always requires professional investigation.

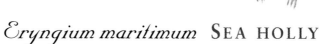

Eryngium maritimum

Filipendula ulmaria MEADOWSWEET

Growing in abundance on banks and ditches across the British Isles, Europe and temperate Asia, meadowsweet produces tufts of small, fragrant creamy-white flowers. The flowering herb contains tannins, salicylates and a volatile oil.

Actions Meadowsweet is anti-inflammatory, antiseptic, antipyretic and diaphoretic. When used topically it is also rubefacient and analgesic.

Uses Meadowsweet has long been used for urinary infections, to induce sweating in high fevers and for infantile diarrhoea. It is a stomachic herb, good for acid indigestion and heartburn – in contrast to aspirin, which derives from it but can irritate the stomach lining. Meadowsweet is widely used as an anti-inflammatory herb for arthritis and rheumatism.

Dosage and preparations
For rheumatic conditions large doses are needed:
Tincture – 1:1, 25%, 5 ml.
Infusion – a daily dose of 50 g.
For other conditions:
Tincture – 1:5, 25%, 1–2 ml.
Infusion – 1 g per cup, steeped for 5 minutes.

Cautions and contraindications
Do not use if there is kidney damage or in conjunction with anti-inflammatory drugs or anticoagulant therapy.

Filipendula ulmaria

Foeniculum vulgare FENNEL

An erect biennial that thrives on dry soils in Mediterranean and temperate regions, producing umbrella-type spokes of yellow flowers from July to October. The thread-like leaves are much used as a condiment, especially with fish, and the root is a very aromatic salad vegetable. The seeds (strictly speaking the fruits) are used medicinally and as a condiment and digestive. They contain a volatile oil which includes anethole, also found in aniseed, and some related compounds with oestrogenic properties which act like the female hormone oestrogen that is found naturally in the body.

Actions Relaxing and warming to the digestive system, fennel is also a mild antidepressant and a gentle bronchodilator that relieves asthma. Anethole is structurally similar to some of the major mood-regulating neurotransmitters in the brain. It is galactagogue and emmenagogue. The medieval herbalist Hildegarde of Bingen regarded fennel as an all-purpose herb that promoted good health.

Uses Relieves debility and lethargy together with depression, poor digestion and flatulence. It is a gentle expectorant, mainly used for children. Fennel is excellent for nursing mothers, increasing the flow of breast milk and, as the volatile substances are passed through the breast milk, helps to relieve colic in babies.

Dosage and preparations
Tincture – 1:5, 45%, 1–2 ml.
Infusion – 2–4 g of seeds per cup.

Cautions and contraindications
Do not take high doses for long periods.

Foeniculum vulgare

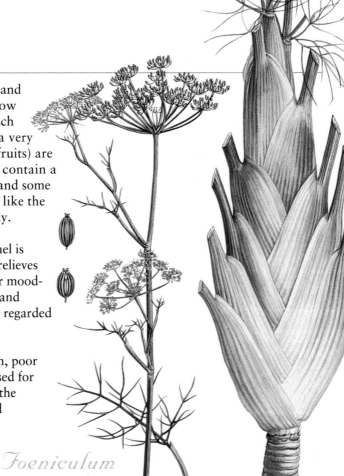

Fucus vesiculosus BLADDERWRACK

The thallus, or frond, of this common seaweed, also known as kelp, is gathered in early to mid-summer and then dried rapidly. It contains minerals, most notably iodine, a wide range of trace elements including chromium, and polysaccharides (mucilage).

Actions Kelp has been used since the 18th century to treat goitre, a swollen, underactive thyroid gland, as the thyroid requires iodine to make its hormone, thyroxine. Kelp has also been long used – and clinically proven to help – in the treatment of obesity. There are probably several reasons for this. Kelp helps to stimulate the thyroid, while the presence of chromium helps to prevent the accumulation of fat.

Uses Helpful in the treatment of obesity and thyroid underactivity (under professional supervision), kelp is also used as a bulking agent to relieve colic and constipation and as a traditional remedy for arthritic stiffness and pain.

Dosage and preparations
Take up to 2 g of dried herb or fresh equivalent daily in a tea, tincture, decoction or as tablets.

Cautions and contraindications
Weight loss with the aid of herbs should be attempted only under professional supervision. Although kelp is a balanced, gentle remedy, excessive amounts may over-stimulate the thyroid gland, putting a strain on the heart.

Fucus vesiculosus

Galium aparine CLEAVERS

An angular, rough and hairy plant, with leaves in whorls (rings around the stem) and tiny flowers that are followed by hairy fruit. The fruit of cleavers adheres to clothes, fur or hair, giving rise to the old common names of 'sticky willie' or 'sticky jack'. The roasted seeds can be used as a coffee substitute. The aerial parts are gathered in May and June, when coming into flower, and contain glycosides, phenolic acids and tannins.

Actions A mild diuretic, cleavers is believed to relax the urinary vessels, facilitate the passage of small urinary stones, and to help dissolve calcium stones. Cleavers is one of the main remedies for stimulating the lymphatic system, which drains excess fluid and toxins from the body's tissues.

Uses As a tissue cleanser, cleavers is commonly used for skin diseases, particularly psoriasis and arthritis, as well as conditions in which the lymph glands are enlarged. It can be used to drain excess fluid and is a traditional slimming aid. One of the main traditional uses of cleavers was to dissolve or expel kidney stones.

Dosage and preparations
Preparations made from the fresh herb are best.
Tincture – 1:5, 25%, 5–10 ml.
Juice – 5–10 ml, refrigerated or made into ice cubes.

Cautions and contraindications
Safe in normal use – no known contraindications.

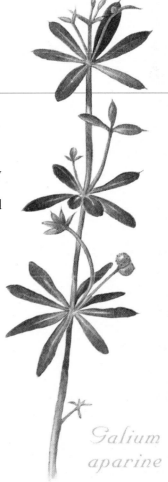

Galium aparine

Gentiana lutea GENTIAN

The main parts used are the root and rhizome of this attractive, medium to tall perennial, which produces clusters of golden flowers in the upper leaf axils. Native to Alpine and upland pastures in central and southern Europe, gentian can be raised from seed in the UK. The root tastes sweet at first, then intensely bitter, due to the presence of bitter glycosides.

Actions A bitter digestive stimulant and anti-inflammatory, the bitter principle increases saliva production and stimulates the appetite and the digestive organs. Gentian is an important ingredient in some aperitifs, taken before a meal to improve appetite and digestion. The bitterness can be tasted at extremely low concentrations, so gentian should be used sparingly to avoid irritation and unpleasant aftertaste.

Uses Gentian is used specifically for loss of appetite, sluggish digestion and elimination and for general debility. It is also useful when taken internally as a cooling herb in high fevers.

Dosage and preparations
Tincture – 1:5, 25%, 10–20 drops an hour before meals. Infusion – 0.5–1 g.

Cautions and contraindications
Some people are very sensitive to bitters and gentian may give them headaches. Gentian is inadvisable for sufferers of stomach and duodenal ulcers.

Gentiana lutea

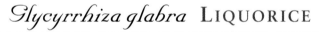

Glycyrrhiza glabra LIQUORICE

Liquorice likes sandy soil and has lived for thousands of years in the flood plains of southeast Europe and southwest Asia. The root and stolons (runners) have been used medicinally for at least 3000 years. They contain glycosides, mucilage and intensely sweet saponins (*glycyrrhiza* means 'sweet root').

Actions Liquorice forms a soothing coating in the stomach and other parts of the digestive tract which encourages mucus production and acts as a soothing expectorant. Antispasmodic and healing, liquorice's saponins, similar to the body's own steroid hormones, increase some hormonal effects. They counteract inflammation and promote water and sodium retention. Liquorice root is also antiviral, notably against the Herpes simplex (cold sore) virus.

Uses Liquorice is a harmonising, soothing tonic that is useful for hot, dry conditions. It is commonly used in prescriptions for arthritis, eczema and asthma, and especially for mouth ulcers, heartburn, gastritis and peptic ulcers (drugs have been developed from it for treating ulcers). It is often used (professionally only) for supporting steroid withdrawal and poor hormone production. Externally it is helpful for cold sores and eczema.

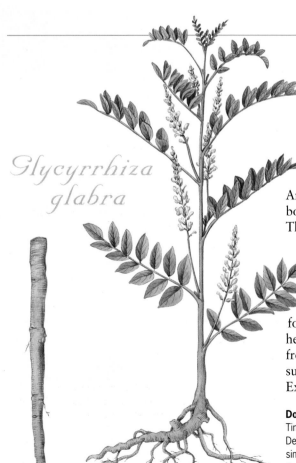

Glycyrrhiza glabra

Dosage and preparations
Tincture – 1:3, 25%, 1–2 ml. Decoction – 1 tablespoon to 600 ml simmered for 20 minutes, or chew the dried root.

Cautions and contraindications
May cause water retention – avoid in the case of high blood pressure. To counteract water retention combine with dandelion leaf and a low-sodium diet.

Hordeum vulgare BARLEY

Barley has been grown as a food crop in the Northern hemisphere for at least 6000 years. Roman gladiators ate it to build up their physical strength and it is a staple across the world. It is a well-balanced food, high in starch, lysine, fibre, calcium, iron, magnesium and potassium.

Actions Extensive research by the Department of Agriculture in the USA has established barley's action to reduce levels of cholesterol in the blood and low density lipoproteins (LDLs). The substances responsible are found mainly in the bran, but also throughout the kernel. Green barley, the juice of young barley leaves, is a concentrated source of vitamins and minerals, and high in superoxide dismutase (SOD), a potent antioxidant which is thought to reduce many of the effects of ageing.

Uses A grain commonly used in bread, flour, soups, stews and sauces, barley helps to prevent heart and circulatory diseases. Green barley is a useful nutritional supplement for preventing or remedying nutritional deficiencies, especially those of iron, magnesium and potassium. It is also an antioxidant with cardio-protective and possibly cancer-preventing properties. Barley and barley malt are nourishing for convalescents. Barley drinks are soothing to intestinal and urinary irritations.

Dosage and preparations
Green barley – a wineglass of the fresh juice morning and night.

Cautions and contraindications
Do not take if suffering from gluten sensitivity.

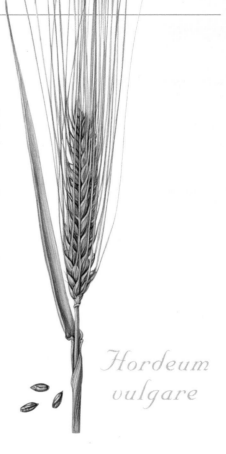

Hordeum vulgare

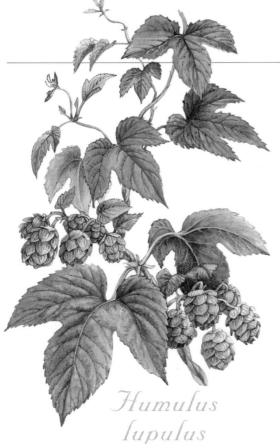

Humulus lupulus

Humulus lupulus HOPS

A tall, climbing perennial, hops were introduced to the UK from mainland Europe for beer-making in the 17th century, after hundreds of years of local resistance to the idea. The clusters of female flowers, used for brewing and for medicine, contain a bitter resin, a volatile oil, flavonoids and an oestrogenic substance.

Actions Many compounds in hops contribute to a sedative action. The bitter resins are strongly antibacterial and anti-inflammatory but degrade fairly quickly in the dried plant, producing a volatile substance which is also sedative.

Uses Relieves irritability and restlessness, especially with insomnia; best combined with other relaxants. Hops are also good for loss of appetite and conditions where bowel rhythm and function are upset. They have a traditional use in treating premature ejaculation and excitability in men, and the sedative effect may be complemented by a hormonal influence brought about by the hops.

Dosage and preparations
Tincture – 1:5, 60%, 1–2 ml.
Infusion – 0.5–1 g per cup.
Should be fairly fresh for digestive properties and can be made into hop pillows when older, as volatile sedative substances accumulate.

Cautions and contraindications
Do not use in cases of depression. Prolonged high doses of hops can cause pustular rashes. Hop pickers report side effects including menstrual irregularities (women), loss of libido (men), fatigue and nausea.

Hydrastis canadensis GOLDENSEAL

A small plant from the USA, liking damp, shaded woodlands, goldenseal is extremely difficult to cultivate. The root is harvested after five years and is usually used powdered but may then be adulterated with barberry bark, a relative. Expense and scarcity make it advisable to use alternatives until it can be grown and harvested more successfully. Goldenseal contains alkaloids, which seem responsible for most of its actions.

Actions Goldenseal is a powerful antiseptic, and is astringent and healing to the gut wall and other mucous membranes. Often included in prescriptions for the lungs, reproductive tract and kidneys, goldenseal is also a bitter digestive stimulant, a liver tonic and cholagogue.

Uses Internally, goldenseal is excellent for catarrhal complaints of all kinds, but as it is cooling in nature, it should be combined with warming remedies such as ginger and cinnamon. It is one of the most widely used herbs for inflammation of the digestive tract and for sinus problems. It is antibacterial and antifungal and an infusion is a useful topical application for thrush.

Dosage and preparations
Tincture – 1:10, 60%, 0.5–2 ml.
Infusion – up to 1 g.

Cautions and contraindications
Do not give to children and always take in small doses (due to the alkaloids).

Hydrastis canadensis

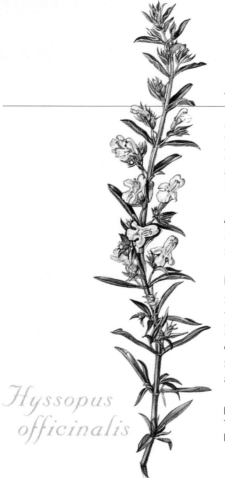

Hyssopus officinalis HYSSOP

An upright herb growing to 1.5 m (5 ft), hyssop produces spikes of blue-violet flowers and spear-shaped leaves which are harvested at the same time. It is a native of the light dry soils of southern Europe and has a strongly aromatic odour and taste. Hyssop is rich in volatile oil and also contains a bitter substance, resin and gum.

Actions Hyssop is sedative, diaphoretic, relaxing and expectorant. Research has demonstrated that hyssop has both an action that soothes the mucous membranes and expectorant properties.

Uses Hippocrates recommended hyssop for chest complaints and it is useful for colds, chest infections, bronchial congestion and asthma. For tight, dry, wheezy coughs combine it with marshmallow or coltsfoot. It is an excellent herb for children, specifically for overexcitability and asthma with a nervous component. A hyssop infusion is relaxing and makes a very pleasant tea for nervous exhaustion. The essential oil, applied diluted, has an antiviral effect and is especially effective against the herpes simplex virus.

Dosage and preparations
Tincture – 1:5, 45%, 1–2 ml.
Infusions – 1–2 g.

Cautions and contraindications
Avoid during pregnancy or with high blood pressure. The oil contains ketones, organic compounds, which are neurotoxic (poisonous to the nervous system). In normal use, risk is minimal.

Hyssopus officinalis

Hypericum perforatum ST JOHN'S WORT

St John's wort is a heathland shrub that grows widely in the UK, Europe and western Asia. It is distinguishable from many of its close relatives by its small oval leaves which are punctured by translucent dots. The leaves and flowers are harvested in summer. Surprisingly, the yellow flowers yield a deep red oil and the herb also contains flavonoid glycosides and tannins.

Actions In Germany a standardised extract of St John's wort has been extensively used and researched as a herbal antidepressant and it is now among the biggest selling medicines in that country. In clinical trials it has proved as effective for mild to moderate depression as major synthetic drugs, but without their side effects. In the Middle Ages, St John's wort was used as a major wound healer, particularly for deep sword wounds. It promotes tissue regeneration and is antibacterial, astringent and antispasmodic. Hypericin, the red pigment found particularly in the oil, is thought to have an antiviral action, and is under investigation as a treatment for HIV infection.

Uses The main use of St John's wort has been in the treatment of moderate depression, and it has been found so effective that the mood-lifting effects become apparent after only a fortnight of treatment. Herbalists prescribe St John's wort more as a nervous system restorative than as simply an antidepressant, however, and use it for many conditions associated with nervous stress – insomnia, anxiety, bedwetting and colic. St John's wort can be of great benefit in treating menopausal complaints such as mood swings, irritability and low energy. St John's wort's antispasmodic and relaxing effects make it a useful herb for digestive complaints marked by nervous tension. Externally, the oil's healing and mild analgesic properties help to ease the pain caused by arthritis, neuralgia (nerve irritation) and shingles, and help to soothe burns and wounds.

Dosage and preparations
Tincture – 1:5, 45%, 2–4 ml.
Infusion – 2–5 g per cup.
To make the infused oil collect the flowers in June or July and pack them into a jar containing sunflower oil. Leave on a sunny windowsill for at least a fortnight and then press out and filter the oil, which will have turned a deep red colour because of the hypericin in it.

Cautions and contraindications
The use of St John's wort, especially externally, can trigger temporary photosensitive (sensitivity to sunlight) skin rashes. If this occurs, stop taking the St John's wort until the rash has subsided and avoid exposure to sunlight on subsequent occasions when taking the herb.

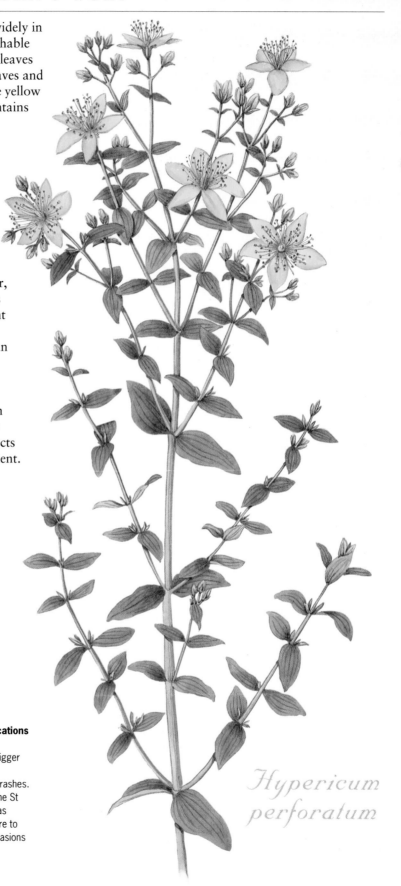

Hypericum perforatum

Inula helenium ELECAMPANE

A large herb, growing up to 3 m (10 ft), elecampane is native to central Europe and Asia. The rhizomes of two or three-year-old plants are usually collected in spring or autumn. They contain both a volatile oil and a bitter principle and are dried at low temperature because the volatile oil is easily lost. Elecampane has a distinctive, aromatic flavour and was a common ingredient in many digestive liqueurs and old-fashioned cough candies.

Actions Elecampane is expectorant, antitussive and supports digestive and eliminatory functions. Certain components of the essential oil stimulate the tissues of the digestive tract, which in turn stimulate a reflex in the respiratory and urinary systems. This stimulation and reflex help to liquefy secretions, thus aiding elimination of waste.

Uses Excellent for relieving chronic, catarrhal coughs, particularly in the elderly, elecampane is also useful for relieving digestive debility and was traditionally used as an anthelmintic. It is also used externally for scabies, herpes and other skin infections and infestation.

Dosage and preparations
Best prepared fresh.
Tincture – 1:5, 45%, 2–4 ml.
Infusion/cold decoction – 1–3 g per cup.

Cautions and contraindications
Avoid use during pregnancy and lactation. Elecampane can cause sensitising and allergic reactions of the skin. Large doses must be avoided as they can cause vomiting, diarrhoea and spasms.

Inula helenium

Juniperus communis JUNIPER

An evergreen shrub often seen on exposed heathland slanting away from the prevailing wind, juniper is widely distributed throughout the Northern Hemisphere and common in the northern UK. The berries are harvested from September to October and are used as a flavouring for gin as well as for their medicinal properties.

Actions Juniper is diuretic, antiseptic – especially for the urinary tract – assists elimination of uric acid and is a relaxing digestive tonic. External applications stimulate the circulation.

Uses A powerful urinary antiseptic for cystitis and a stimulating cleanser for rheumatism, tendon problems, gout and neuralgia. Externally the diluted essential oil is an excellent rub or bath for tight muscles and rheumatic pain.

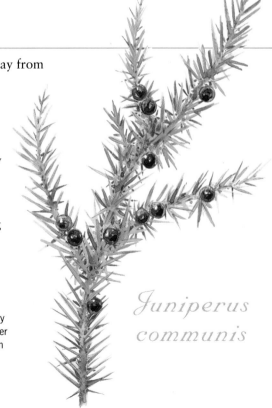

Dosage and preparations
Tincture – 1:5, 45%, 1–2 ml.
A few berries can be eaten raw or infused, fresh or dried.
For external use the essential oil may be mixed up to 5% in a base oil. Infused oil can be made by macerating 100 g of crushed berries in 1 litre of oil for 15 days, in sunlight.

Cautions and contraindications
Do not use if suffering from a kidney disease or during pregnancy. Juniper has an old and unjustified reputation for being toxic to the kidneys, but recent research shows it to be completely safe in normal doses.

Juniperus communis

Laurus nobilis BAY

Bay can grow to a height of 20 m (60 ft), but in the UK rarely exceeds 8 m (25 ft) and is often grown as an ornamental tree as well as a pot herb. The leaves are popular as a flavouring for sauces and the oil is sometimes used in perfumery.

Actions The oil of the bay tree has antiseptic, antifungal and stimulant properties.

Uses The infused oil makes an excellent rub for general aches and pains, rheumatic complaints, sprains and bruises. A tincture of the berries in rum (bay rum) is a traditional stimulating application for improving hair condition.

Dosage and preparations
One or two leaves used in stews and soups to strengthen digestion. Tincture – 1:5, 45%, applied topically.

Cautions and contraindications
Contact dermatitis may occasionally result from handling the essential oil. If you are picking your own bay leaves be sure you have the correct species. The cherry laurel (*Prunus laurocerasus*), looks very similar but is poisonous.

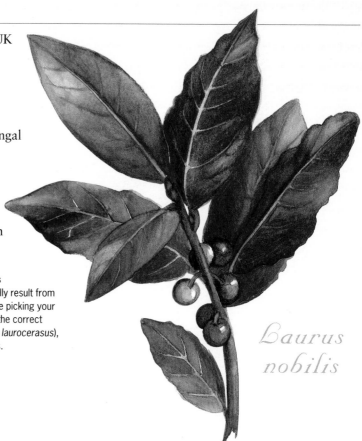

Laurus nobilis

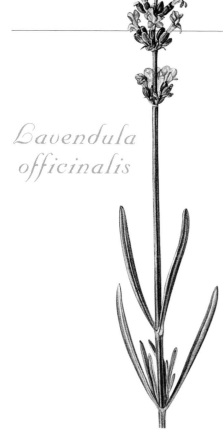

Lavendula officinalis

Lavendula officinalis LAVENDER

Native to southern Europe, lavender is popular as a border or hedging plant in gardens for its flowers, its attraction for bees and its pleasing smell. The flowers contain tannins and a gentle essential oil.

Actions A sedative and antidepressant, lavender is also carminative, mildly spasmolytic and cholagogue. The volatile oil is anti-infective, rubefacient, antirheumatic and healing, especially for burns. It is also sedative when applied to the skin and very effective in a bath.

Uses The infusion or tincture is useful for excitability, headaches, nervous palpitations and insomnia. It is also very helpful for colic and for digestive problems of a nervous origin. The volatile oil, as long as it is of good quality, is both healing and disinfecting, making it extremely useful for burns, fungal skin disorders and other skin infections. You can also use it externally or in an oil vaporiser for respiratory infections and for ear infections in children, if the drum is not perforated.

Dosage and preparations
Tincture – 1:5, 45%, up to 2 ml.
Infusions can be used topically (10 g) or internally (1–2 g).
Infused oil – make in a sealed, transparent container and leave in sunlight for a week.
Essential oil – dilute to 10–25%. May be applied neat to burns.

Cautions and contraindications
High doses may cause excitation or headaches.

Leonurus cardiaca MOTHERWORT

This dark green, bushy plant, with toothed leaves and whorls (rings) of pale pink flowers, is found in hedgerows across temperate regions. Motherwort has a traditional use in midwifery at childbirth to increase contractions. It contains alkaloids and bitter glycosides.

Actions Motherwort is a gentle uterine stimulant and relaxant. Modern research has indicated possible effects in calming the heart and lowering blood pressure.

Uses Motherwort has three spheres of influence: nervous, circulatory and uterine. It is used for delayed, painful or irregular menstruation, especially associated with nervous tension or at the menopause. Motherwort is traditionally used to treat palpitations and is helpful for the nervous or hormonal problems that may underlie this complaint in women. It is best, however, to seek professional help, as palpitations occasionally indicate heart problems for which motherwort may not be adequate treatment.

Dosage and preparations
Tincture – 1:5, 25%, 2–5 ml.
Infusion – 2–4 g per cup.

Cautions and contraindications
Do not use during pregnancy, except under the instruction of a qualified midwife.

Leonurus cardiaca

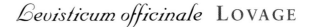

Levisticum officinale LOVAGE

Levisticum officinale

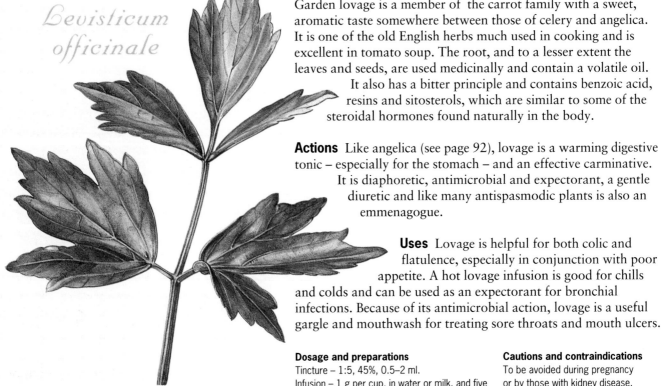

Garden lovage is a member of the carrot family with a sweet, aromatic taste somewhere between those of celery and angelica. It is one of the old English herbs much used in cooking and is excellent in tomato soup. The root, and to a lesser extent the leaves and seeds, are used medicinally and contain a volatile oil. It also has a bitter principle and contains benzoic acid, resins and sitosterols, which are similar to some of the steroidal hormones found naturally in the body.

Actions Like angelica (see page 92), lovage is a warming digestive tonic – especially for the stomach – and an effective carminative. It is diaphoretic, antimicrobial and expectorant, a gentle diuretic and like many antispasmodic plants is also an emmenagogue.

Uses Lovage is helpful for both colic and flatulence, especially in conjunction with poor appetite. A hot lovage infusion is good for chills and colds and can be used as an expectorant for bronchial infections. Because of its antimicrobial action, lovage is a useful gargle and mouthwash for treating sore throats and mouth ulcers.

Dosage and preparations
Tincture – 1:5, 45%, 0.5–2 ml.
Infusion – 1 g per cup, in water or milk, and five times that strength as a mouthwash or gargle.

Cautions and contraindications
To be avoided during pregnancy or by those with kidney disease.

Mahonia aquifolium OREGON GRAPE

Oregon grape is a purple-berried shrub with holly-shaped leaves that is native to the western coast of the USA. Elsewhere it is a popular garden plant.

Actions Oregon grape can be used as a tissue cleanser, an alterative and a digestive stimulant. Recent research has shown that it can inhibit some types of lipid breakdown in the body which contribute to inflammation in psoriasis. It may also be an important antifungal agent for the gut, due to the action of the alkaloid berberine.

Uses Oregon grape is a useful herb for chronic skin, joint and other inflammatory problems and it should be used topically for psoriasis. It has long had a reputation as one of the main alterative or cleansing herbs and is a staple in prescriptions for eczema and psoriasis. Recently Oregon grape has been used to treat fungal overgrowth in the gut and other conditions associated with this. Oregon grape's bitter and cholagogue effects are useful for poor appetite, sluggish digestion and poor liver function.

Mahonia aquifolium

Dosage and preparations
Tincture – 1:5, 25%, 2–4 ml.
Decoction – 1–2 g per cup simmered for 20 minutes.

Cautions and contraindications
Do not take during pregnancy.

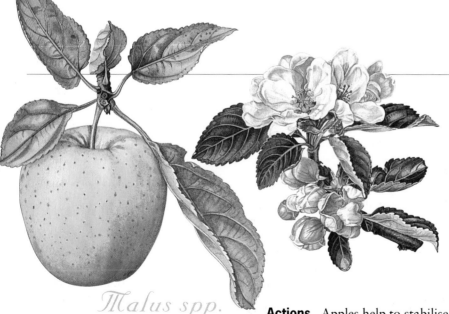

Malus spp.

Malus spp. APPLE

Apple trees grow throughout Europe and were probably introduced to the UK by the Romans. Apples are a very healthy food, as folk wisdom has always held, and eating two apples a day over several weeks has been shown to reduce levels of cholesterol. It also appears to shift the profile of lipids in the blood away from the dangerous low density types (LDL) to the safer high density ones (HDL). This is particularly true for many people with a genetic tendency to high cholesterol and, for some unknown reason, for women.

Dosage and preparations
To make the most of all the beneficial effects of apples they are best eaten fresh and unpeeled. Apples should be washed carefully before eating.

Cautions and contraindications
Unripe or unpeeled apples can exacerbate chronic diarrhoea in children and irritable bowel syndrome in some adults.

Actions Apples help to stabilise blood sugar, providing sustained release of sugars in the blood, without the sudden rise followed by an insulin surge and low blood sugar usually caused by eating sweet foods. The polyphenols which are concentrated in and under the peel are antiviral and may help reduce the risk of some cancers.

Uses Apples are also helpful to the digestion in regulating bowel movements and are traditionally believed to aid the digestion of fatty foods, hence the custom of serving apple sauce with roast pork.

Melissa officinalis LEMON BALM

This familiar, lemon-scented garden herb is a favourite with bees. The herb is harvested just before flowering and in the early afternoon, when the volatile oil content peaks, and is best used fresh. Other than the volatile oil, lemon balm contains tannins and a bitter principle.

Actions Lemon balm is a relaxant with antispasmodic, carminative and mildly diaphoretic properties. It has been used 'to make the heart merry' since ancient times. Clinical trials have clearly demonstrated lemon balm's ability to calm nervous tension, probably due to the absorption of the volatile oil by emotional centres in the mid-brain. Hot water extracts have antiviral, antihistamine, antispasmodic activity and the diluted essential oil helps to relieve the pain of shingles.

Uses An excellent herb for restlessness, agitation and irritability especially associated with neuralgia, headaches, palpitations or gastric upset. Take plentifully after a meal as a relaxing digestive and before bed to prevent insomnia and nightmares.

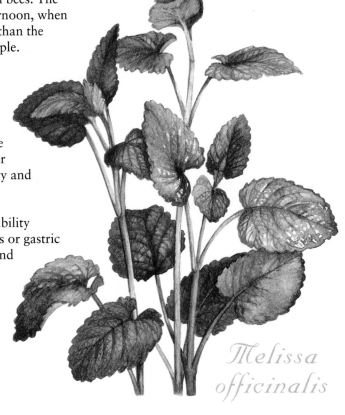

Melissa officinalis

Dosage and preparations
Tincture – 1:5, 45%, 2–5 ml.
Infusion – 2–4 g or 2 fresh leaves per cup. For shingles or neuralgia, use 5% essential oil in a cream or base oil.

Cautions and contraindications
Lemon balm is a safe herb to use and very well suited to children.

Mentha x piperita PEPPERMINT

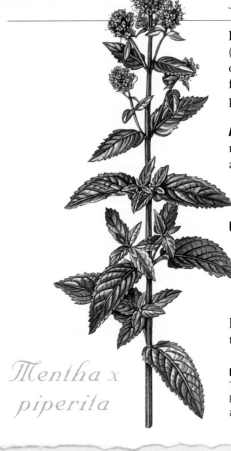

Mentha x piperita

Peppermint is a hybrid of water mint (*Mentha aquatica*) and spearmint (*Mentha x spicata*), which has been used medicinally since at least the time of the Ancient Egyptians. The leaves are harvested just before the plant flowers and contain a volatile oil rich in menthol, together with flavonoids, phenolic acids, tannin-like substances and a bitter principle.

Actions Peppermint is an aromatic digestive stimulant; the flavonoids are mildly antispasmodic and the oil is powerfully antispasmodic, carminative and choleretic. Peppermint oil is strongly antibacterial, antiprotozoal and drying when inhaled. Topically, it is cooling and anaesthetic when very dilute but in higher concentration causes heat and redness.

Uses Peppermint is a useful remedy for colic, diarrhoea, sluggish digestion, flatulence and the relief of nausea. A hot infusion helps to relieve colds and bronchitis and the essential oil can be inhaled for congested catarrh. At concentrations of 0.5–1 per cent, the oil soothes painful and itchy eczema, neuralgia, shingles, psoriasis and rheumatic pain.
Water mint has similar properties to peppermint. Spearmint, a favourite of kitchen gardens, is helpful for easing digestive upsets associated with nervous tension, having a gentler action than peppermint.

Dosage and preparations
Tincture – 1:5, 45%, 10–20 drops.
Infusion – 2–4 g per cup, between and after meals.

Cautions and contraindications
Use as an inhalant for short periods only and do not use for babies. Avoid in heartburn. Do not use the essential oil during pregnancy.

Ocimum basilicum BASIL

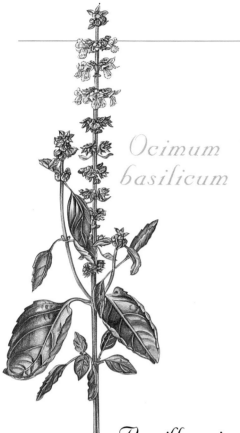

Ocimum basilicum

Basil is now used mainly for cooking, but for many centuries it was a very important medicinal plant across the world. It is a non-hardy plant that grows in warm climates and likes a sunny position. The medicinal properties lie in the leaves, which contain a volatile oil and vitamins A and C.

Actions Basil is a nervous restorative and antidepressant. It is mildly sedative and is a reputed stimulant for the adrenal system which regulates hormone levels. The volatile oil is strongly anti-infective, and has a decongestant and antispasmodic action. It can also be used as a carminative and a galactogogue and is an aromatic, digestive stimulant with some vermicidal activity.

Uses Inhalations of the essential oil are useful for clearing and disinfecting the sinuses and air passages during head colds and chest infections. Basil is a useful herb to take when depressed or in low spirits and combines well with lemon balm. It is also used to improve sluggish digestion and encourage milk production in nursing mothers.

Dosage and preparations
Basil is more effective in the form of a tincture, (1:5, 45%, 1–3 ml), than as an infusion. The fresh leaves (far superior to the dried) can be eaten regularly in salads as a nerve tonic – 1–3 leaves per day will suffice.

Cautions and contraindications
Pregnant women should avoid medicinal doses of basil. Culinary amounts should not interfere with pregnancy but, if in doubt, avoid.

Passiflora incarnata PASSIONFLOWER

Passionflower is a native of the USA. Its aerial parts are collected for medicinal use after the edible passion fruits have been harvested. The first recorded medicinal use of passionflower was in the USA in 1867, but it only became a popular element in European herbal medicine in the 1920s. The herb contains useful alkaloids and flavonoids.

Actions Passionflower has a mild sedative effect, thought to derive from its flavonoids, which have some of the same pharmacological effects as the widely used prescription sedative, diazepam, but without the side effects. Its anodyne and antispasmodic properties are thought to be derived from other constituents.

Uses Passionflower is one of the most popular herbs for the self-treatment of neuralgia, restlessness, irritability, excitability and insomnia. Although passionflower is not always strong enough to use by itself for encouraging sleep, it is useful in supporting the actions of other sedatives, such as hops and valerian. Although only based on animal studies, the influential and ongoing German Commission E report into herbal remedies recommends passionflower for nervous restlessness. Passionflower has also been found to give partial relief from the pain of shingles.

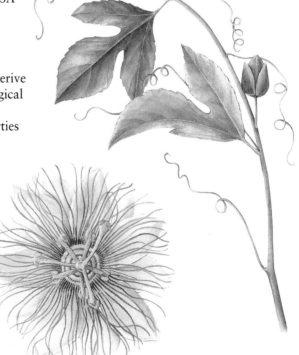

Passiflora incarnata

Dosage and preparations
Tincture – 1:5, 25%, 2–4 ml.
Infusion – 1 g per cup steeped for 5 minutes.

Cautions and contraindications.
None known.

Petroselinum crispum PARSLEY

Indigenous to the eastern Mediterranean, parsley has been widely cultivated since the time of the ancient Greeks to the present day and flourishes in a sunny position and rich, limey soil. Two-year-old roots and leaves are used medicinally and contain volatile oil, flavonoids, vitamins A and C, and iron, calcium, phosphorus and manganese.

Actions Parsley is diuretic, nutritive, carminative and antispasmodic. It is also a stomachic and general stimulant to the digestive organs, as well as being a useful breath freshener.

Uses Parsley is very useful for relieving water retention and its digestive stimulating properties make it a good general cleanser for congested conditions. It is indicated in anaemia and nutritional deficiency because of its mineral content and is excellent for poor appetite and digestion and for flatulence and colic. A sprig of parsley is also very effective for reducing garlic breath.

Dosage and preparations
Tincture – 1:5, 45%, 2–5 ml.
Infusion – 2 g per cup, covered and steeped for 5 minutes.
Decoction of root – 3–4 g per cup covered and simmered for 20 minutes. For nutritional deficiency, add sprigs of fresh parsley to salads.

Cautions and contraindications
Avoid taking parsley during pregnancy and if you are suffering from any form of kidney disease. Parsley seeds are strongly diuretic but somewhat toxic; avoid them.

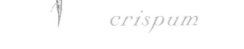

Petroselinum crispum

Phytolacca americana POKEROOT

Pokeroot is a strikingly tall perennial which produces drooping clusters of red berries. It is indigenous to the eastern USA, but has become naturalised in Europe and prefers damp, shady conditions. The dried root contains saponins, alkaloids and resins.

Actions Pokeroot has a long-standing reputation as a powerful lymphatic alterative and stimulant. It also stimulates elimination and possibly has an action that stimulates white blood cell activity.

Uses Pokeroot was an important herb for the shamanistic practitioners of North America in the last century, who used it for a wide range of infectious and congestive disorders. It is now used mainly for relieving swollen lymph nodes and conditions affecting lymphatic and glandular tissues, such as mumps, tonsillitis and swollen adenoids; as a tissue cleanser for rheumatic and chronic skin complaints; and as an aid to weight loss, where it has gained a reputation for helping to break down fat. Applied topically, pokeroot is a helpful tincture for acne and poultice for mastitis.

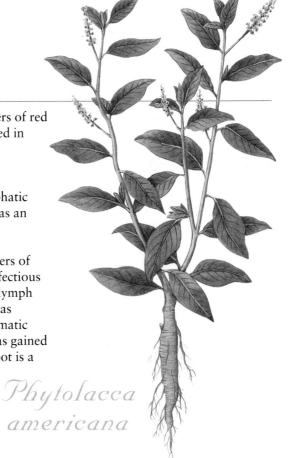

Phytolacca americana

Dosage and preparations
Tincture – 1:5, 25%, 5–10 drops.
Decoction – 0.5 g per day, simmered in a cup of water for 20 minutes.

Cautions and contraindications
Pokeroot should not be used during pregnancy and is not suitable for self-treatment or in large doses – it can be irritant, emetic and cathartic.

Plantago spp. PLANTAIN (PSYLLIUM)

Plantain is a low to medium-sized hardy perennial with single stems that bear a spike of tiny grey-brown flowers. The leaves are gathered during the flowering period. It is widely distributed around the Northern Hemisphere, in grasslands and by fresh water, and is very difficult to eradicate from lawns. Plantain was much used by the Anglo-Saxons as a laxative and for bites and wounds, and contains mucilage, tannins and minerals such as zinc, silica and potassium.

Plantago spp.

Actions Plantain is laxative, mildly astringent and healing with styptic and demulcent properties. Ribwort plantain is widely used by herbalists as an anticatarrhal tonic for mucous membranes and a relaxing expectorant.

Uses Plantain is an excellent restorative and tonic for all forms of respiratory congestion – nasal catarrh, bronchitis, sinusitis and middle ear infections. Plantain's demulcent quality makes it useful for painful urination. Topically it calms the irritation and itching of insect bites, stings and skin irritations. It is also an effective laxative and a disinfectant and styptic for wounds.

Dosage and preparations
Tincture – 1:5, 25%, 2–5 ml.
Infusion – 2–3 g per cup, infused for 5 minutes.
Fresh juice or tincture are styptic but this property is inactivated by heating.

Cautions and contraindications
None known.

Rheum palmatum CHINESE RHUBARB

Chinese rhubarb is indigenous to the hilly areas of central and eastern Asia and was introduced to the UK in the 18th century. The culinary use of the stalks was a late development as mainly the root was used – taken as a form of laxative. Rhubarb root contains anthraquinones (which are strongly laxative), tannins and bitters.

Actions In very small doses an astringent digestive tonic, stimulating liver and gall-bladder function, but in larger doses rhubarb is purgative.

Uses Chinese rhubarb should be taken for a sluggish digestion and diarrhoea in small doses and for occasional constipation in larger doses. It has been used to treat bacterial dysentery, perhaps by stimulating the body's natural means of ridding itself of the bacteria or because of the effect of the tannins, which are antibacterial. English rhubarb *(Rheum officinale)* is also used and is a tonic for oestrogen deficiency, particularly for women during the menopause.

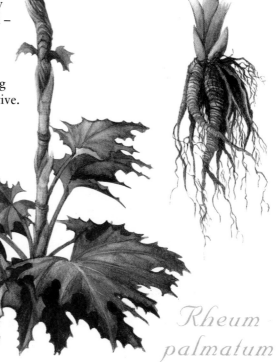

Rheum palmatum

Dosage and preparations
Tincture – 1:5, 25%, 0.5–4 ml.
Powder – 0.1–1 g daily.

Cautions and contraindications
You should not take rhubarb during pregnancy or if you are suffering from gout or arthritis. Also refrain from using it if bowel obstruction is suspected or localised abdominal pain is present. The leaves are poisonous.

Rosa spp ROSE

Cultivated roses were originally native to the eastern Mediterranean, where they were widespread in decorative, ceremonial and symbolic use more than 2500 years ago, but are now popular worldwide. Their medicinal properties reside mainly in the sweet, intensely fragrant oil containing nerol, geraniol and other constituents. Dog rose is widespread in the temperate regions of both hemispheres, and vitamin C was first discovered in its fruit – rosehips. Rosehips also contain tannins, flavonoids and mucilage.

Actions The petals of roses have antispasmodic, sedative and astringent properties. They are locally antiseptic and a gentle laxative. They can also help to regulate the menstrual cycle and are anti-inflammatory. Rosewater is a gentle skin cleanser and the basis of a skin-protective cold cream. Rosehip tea can be used to relieve and treat scurvy and is mildly astringent and diuretic.

Uses Rosehip tea is an old folk remedy for colds and mild diarrhoea. Rose petals make a pleasant, soothing and anti-inflammatory infusion, which is helpful for digestive debility, respiratory and gastrointestinal infestations, and poor concentration. It can also alleviate depression and anxiety and be taken for irregular or heavy periods. The oil – which is very expensive and only worth using if unadulterated – also reduces inflammation and fights fungal infection.

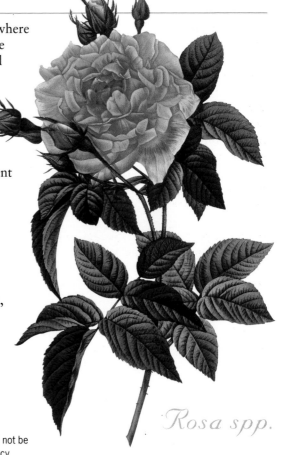

Rosa spp.

Dosage and preparations
Infusion – petals 1 g per cup. Fresh petals give best results.

Cautions and contraindications
Petals and oil should not be used during pregnancy.

Rosmarinus officinalis ROSEMARY

This aromatic kitchen herb thrives on sandy soil in open sunlight and is indigenous to maritime regions of southern Europe. In addition to its volatile oil, rosemary contains flavonoids, a bitter principle and a resin. It has historical associations with remembrance and fidelity. Sprigs of rosemary were traditionally exchanged in a gesture of friendship, thrown into graves in commemoration and worn in the hair to sharpen recollection.

Actions Rosemary is a stimulating tonic, increasing blood flow to the peripheries of the body and the brain, whilst also strengthening capillary walls. It is warming and drying and helps to stimulate the circulation whilst being antispasmodic. Externally it has an anodyne effect on muscle and joint rheumatism; internally it is an aromatic digestive stimulant, increasing the flow of bile. Rosemary is strongly antibacterial and antifungal.

Uses Rosemary is good for depression and debility, especially that associated with nervous tension, particularly when combined with lavender and taken internally or in a bath. It is also useful for migraines and tension headaches that are relieved by heat, and for indigestion, poor appetite and flatulence. Used as a hair rinse, the infusion relieves dandruff and hair loss.

Rosmarinus officinalis

Dosage and preparations
Tincture – 1:5, 45%, 1–3 ml.
Infusion – 2–4 g of dried herb, used mainly in combination with other herbs.

Cautions and contraindications
Avoid during pregnancy – rosemary is a strong uterine stimulant.

Rubus idaeus RASPBERRY

Raspberry grows wild in much of Europe and the UK, and particularly well in Scotland. It likes a rich, loamy soil and can be cultivated by planting suckers 60–90 cm (2–3 ft) apart, with about 1.5 m (4–5 ft) gaps between rows. The leaves contain tannins and an alkaloid and the fruit is rich in vitamin C and minerals.

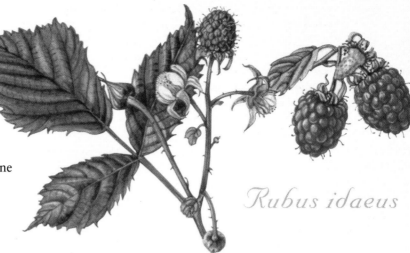

Rubus idaeus

Actions Astringent and toning to the uterine and pelvic muscles.

Uses Raspberry leaf tea is famous for preparing the uterus for childbirth as it increases the strength of contractions and results in easier childbirth. For this purpose the tea should be taken 2 or 3 times daily in the last 3 months of pregnancy. Traditionally it was combined with motherwort (see page 112) for threatened miscarriage. As an astringent remedy, the infusion is a useful treatment for diarrhoea in children. It can also be used as a gargle or mouthwash for mouth ulcers, oral thrush, sore throats and tonsillitis, or as a lotion for nappy rash.

Dosage and preparations
Tincture – 1:5, 25%, 5-10 ml.
Infusion – 5 to 8 g per cup.

Cautions and contraindications
None known.

Salix alba WILLOW

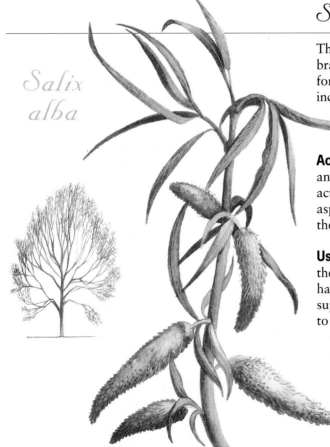

Salix alba

The dried bark of this common tree is collected from young branches during the growth period. Willow bark is famous for containing aspirin-like substances – phenolic glycosides, including salicylates. It also contains flavonoids and tannins. Being very strong and supple, willow twigs have many domestic uses.

Actions Willow is anti-inflammatory, analgesic, antipyretic, antirheumatic and astringent. Interestingly, some of willow's active constituents, while sharing the pain-relieving effects of aspirin (acetylsalicylic acid), have a more sustained action in the body and fewer side effects than aspirin.

Uses Willow bark helps to reduce high fevers and to relieve the pain of arthritis and headaches. Although these claims have not been proven clinically, the indications are strongly supported by the fact that the bark was used in a similar way to aspirin long before the invention of the drug.

Dosage and preparations
Tincture – 1:5, 25%, up to 8 ml.
Decoction – 3–5 g per cup.

Cautions and contraindications
Safe in normal use.

Sambucus nigra ELDER

The elder is a small tree or shrub that grows in woods and on wasteland. It has stiff, pithy stems, producing flat heads of small creamy flowers in June, which give out a characteristic sweet, perfumed smell, and black berries in late summer and early autumn. Elder has a great number of folklore associations. It features, for example, in Arthurian tales, while a Biblical legend holds that Judas hanged himself on the elder tree. Elder has long been associated with witchcraft and religion, which may partly reflect the wide range of medicinal uses of many parts of the plant. It is widely available and has a distinctive look. The flowers and berries are the most commonly used of the shrub's many medicinal parts.

Sambucus nigra

Actions The flowers and berries of the elder are diaphoretic and expectorant. Elderflowers are used in particular to relieve catarrh and to improve the tone of nasal membranes. According to Dr Fritz Weiss, the much respected German herbalist, elderflowers raise the resistance to respiratory infections. Recent laboratory tests in Israel showed that elderberry extract inhibits various strains of the influenza virus and, if taken early on in influenza infection, can dramatically improve recovery times. Both the berries and the flowers encourage the fever response and stimulate sweating, which prevents very high temperatures and provides an important channel for detoxification. In addition the flowers are diuretic, while the berries are mildly laxative. The inner bark has a history of use as a purgative dating back to the time of Hippocrates.

Uses Traditional winter cold remedies using elder include elderberry wine, which should be taken hot and mixed with cinnamon; elderberry rob – a syrup made by simmering down 2.5 kg (5 lb) of elderberries with 500 g (1 lb) of sugar; and elderflowers combined in a hot infusion with peppermint and yarrow. The trick is to take them hot and then rest in order to 'sweat it out'. Elder leaves make a useful ointment for bruises, sprains and wounds. An ointment made from elder flowers is excellent for chilblains and stimulating local circulation. The flowers make popular hay fever treatments for their anticatarrhal properties and their diuretic effect can also help to reduce fluid congestion.

Dosage and preparations
Tincture – 1:5, 25%, 1–5 ml.
Infusion – 1–3 g per cup, can be taken frequently for colds or flu.

Cautions and contraindications
Do not take the bark during pregnancy.

Salvia officinalis SAGE (RED, PURPLE)

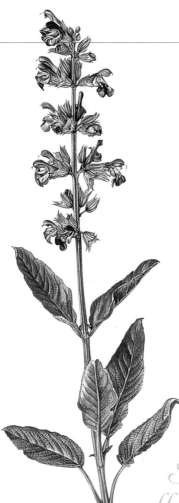

A southern European perennial with purple-green downy leaves and purple flowers, sage is widely grown as a pot herb. The aerial parts are harvested when the flowers are in bud and the small hairs (trichomes) contain a volatile oil. Sage also contains tannins, an oestrogenic principle, a resin and a bitter substance.

Actions Sage powerfully suppresses sweat secretion and milk production and so should be avoided by weaning mothers. It is astringent, antiseptic, aromatic and stomachic. Sage has a long-standing reputation for reducing blood sugar and is traditionally seen as a restorative herb.

Uses Sage is specific for night sweats, hot flushes and symptoms associated with the menopause. It can also be very useful for painful menstruation, stomach problems associated with poor digestion and poor circulation. A tincture or a strong infusion of the fresh herb makes an ideal mouthwash and gargle for mouth ulcers, swollen gums and sore throats. It also makes a good toothpaste.

Dosage and preparations
Tincture – 1:5, 45%, 10–30 drops. Infusion – preferably of the fresh herb, up to 3 g per cup. For hot flushes and night sweats, drink the infusion cold.

Cautions and contraindications
Avoid during pregnancy and breastfeeding. Volatile oil must not be taken internally.

Salvia officinalis

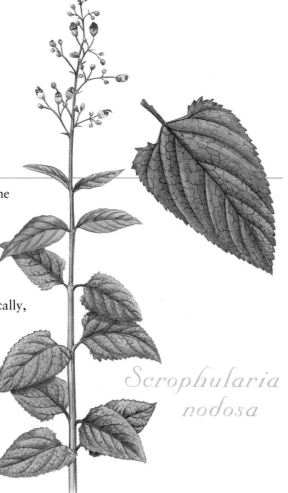

Scrophularia nodosa FIGWORT

A tall, erect perennial with a sharply square stem – one country name for the plant is 'carpenter's square' – figwort grows in moist areas of waste or cultivated ground throughout most of the Northern Hemisphere. Figwort contains saponins, flavonoids and resins.

Actions Figwort is a mild laxative, a lymphatic cleanser and a diuretic. Its mild cardiac stimulatory action may be responsible for its reputation as a stimulant to the lymphatic system. Applied topically, figwort is mildly anodyne.

Uses Figwort is helpful for inflammatory skin conditions, such as eczema and psoriasis, especially where the condition is chronic and there is also discharge or swollen lymph nodes. The bruised leaves were traditionally used as a poultice and topically applied to relieve burns and swellings.

Dosage and preparations
Tincture – 1:5, 25%, 1–3 ml.
Infusion – up to 2 g per cup.

Cautions and contraindications
Should be avoided by sufferers of tachycardia (rapid heartbeat) and other heart conditions.

Scrophularia nodosa

Scutellaria spp. SKULLCAP

Skullcap has distinctive pairs of blue to pink flowers, serrated leaves and seed capsules that look like skullcaps – hence its name. It is found widely across the world in temperate and mountainous tropical regions. Virginia skullcap, (*Scutellaria lateriflora*), is the North American species while (*Scutellaria galericulata*) is favoured in Europe. They both contain a bitter principle, flavonoid glycosides and tannins.

Actions Skullcap is one of the most important herbs currently used to treat the nervous system. It is relaxing, restorative, sedative, anticonvulsive and antispasmodic. It also stimulates and strengthens digestion.

Uses The prime uses of skullcap are for nervous tension with exhaustion and debility, disturbed sleep, depression, fatigue and headaches associated with overwork or worry. These reflect its reputation as the prime relaxing herb used for the nervous system. It has applications as a restorative and antispasmodic for a number of neurological and neuromotor conditions including migraine and the effects of withdrawal from benzodiazepine tranquillisers taken for insomnia. Professionally, skullcap is prescribed to reduce the severity and frequency of epileptic attacks.

Dosage and preparations
Tincture – 1:5, 25%, 2–6 ml.
Infusion – 1–2 g per cup, steeped for 5 minutes.

Cautions and contraindications
No known contraindications. Substitution in commercial samples by wood sage was at one time common and led to a number of reported side effects, giving skullcap an undeserved reputation for toxicity.

Scutellaria spp.

Stellaria media CHICKWEED

A small, soft, trailing annual, chickweed has a light green colour with tiny white flowers and is generally found growing on waste ground, by roadsides and on cultivated ground throughout temperate regions. Lightly boiled, chickweed resembles spring spinach and can be used in salads. It contains anti-inflammatory saponins and mucilage.

Actions Chickweed is a mild expectorant with antipruriginous (anti-itching) and demulcent actions. It calms inflamed and itchy skin conditions.

Uses Chickweed has been used since time immemorial as a poultice and an ointment for inflamed skin conditions, especially where it is accompanied by itching, such as eczema, boils, abscesses and insect bites. It is also a gentle expectorant for productive coughs.

Dosage and preparations
Best used fresh.
Tincture – 1:5, 25%, 3–5 ml.
Infusion – 2–4 g per cup.
For external use an infused oil can be made, or a strong infusion used as a lotion or combined with a cream.

Cautions and contraindications
None known.

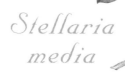

Stellaria media

Stachys officinalis BETONY

Betony is an upright herb with deep reddish-purple flowers. According to Gerard's herbal: 'Betony loves shadowie woods, hedge-rowes, and copses, the borders of pastures, and such like places.' The aerial parts are harvested in July when the herb comes into flower. Betony contains tannins, a bitter principle and alkaloids similar to those in yarrow and vervain.

Actions Betony is mildly diaphoretic and a circulatory stimulant for the head area. It is a general relaxant and restorative to the nervous system and a mild astringent useful in cleaning and drying wounds. Betony is also a gentle digestive and uterine stimulant.

Uses Betony has traditionally been used to treat a huge range of complaints. Augustus Caesar's physician listed no less than 47 diseases for which it was effective. The name is thought to derive from two Celtic words: bew (head) and ton (good). Betony is an excellent herb for sinus congestion and headaches caused by problems in the sinuses and ears. It is also useful for headaches associated with nervous tension or debility.

Betony is a relaxing nervous restorative especially suited to chronic, painful conditions and is useful for relieving chronic insomnia. Hildegard von Bingen (see page 22) recommended betony for people prone to nightmares and it had a long tradition of use in protecting people 'against fearful visions', as Erasmus describes.

Betony can also be used as a cleansing herb, stimulating the liver and the circulation. Alongside its relaxant properties it is an excellent herb for sciatica and rheumatic complaints. It is also a useful tonic for sluggish digestion.

Like yarrow (see page 86), betony was widely used as a herb for wounds. A compress of betony is helpful for minor cuts and bruises and for bites, stings and skin irritations. Also like yarrow, betony can be used to relieve menstrual pain due to congestion associated with slow onset of menses, although it is rarely recommended as a herbal remedy for menstrual complaints.

Dosage and preparations
Tincture – 1:5, 25%, 2–4 ml.
Infusion – 1–3 g per cup.

Cautions and contraindications
Do not take during pregnancy. Large doses may cause diarrhoea and very large doses are emetic.

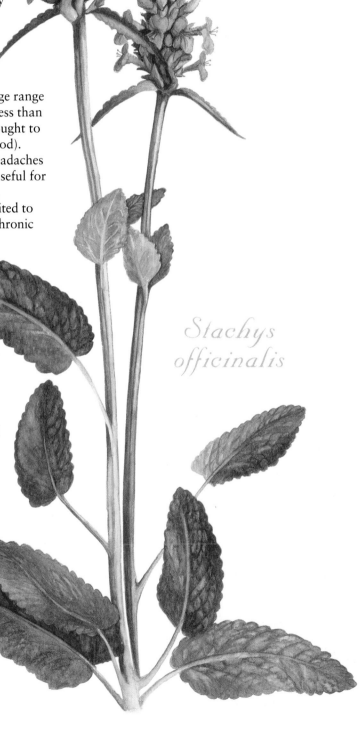

Stachys officinalis

Symphytum officinale COMFREY

A vigorous plant with broad, hairy leaves and bearing drooping spikes of bell-shaped mauve or white flowers, comfrey grows on moist banks and in ditches throughout the UK, Europe and the USA. The leaves and root contain mucilage, tannins and dangerous pyrrolizidine alkaloids.

Actions Comfrey is perhaps the most effective vulnerary herb of all, stimulating the cells which repair skin, connective tissue and bone. It is demulcent and helps to soothe irritation and inflammation in the digestive tract. It is also an astringent and a relaxing expectorant.

Uses Comfrey is excellent applied to shallow wounds, poorly healing skin, strains, sprains and fractures, but should not be used for deep wounds as the surface can heal over too rapidly which may lead to abscesses. Both root and leaf have traditionally been used externally and internally for ulcers, bronchitis and an irritable cough. Due to the problems of toxicity, herbalists currently only use the leaf internally.

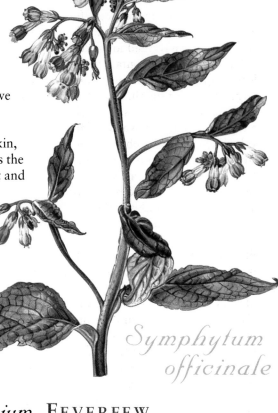

Symphytum officinale

Dosage and preparations
Tincture – (leaf) 1:5, 25%, 2–4 ml.
Infusion – (leaf) 2–3 g per cup.
Leaf and root can be used in ointments and poultices, infused oils and creams.

Cautions and contraindications
Avoid during pregnancy and breast feeding. Do not minister to children under 5 years old. Do not use the root internally. The presence of pyrrolizidine alkaloids, which in isolation can cause liver damage, has raised fears over the safety of comfrey but sensible use of the tea or tincture is quite safe.

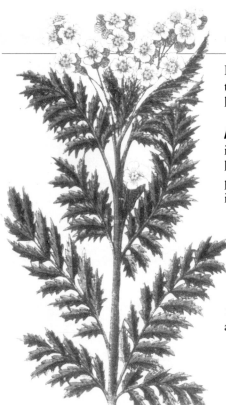

Tanacetum parthenium

Tanacetum parthenium FEVERFEW

Feverfew is a member of the daisy family, which looks like a cross between a tall daisy and camomile. The leaves or aerial parts are harvested when the herb is in flower during the summer months.

Actions Feverfew has anti-inflammatory and diaphoretic actions and helps in the prevention of migraine. The efficacy of feverfew in preventing migraine has been well established. Clinical studies indicate that this action stems, in part, from the regulation of the blood and the regulation of the release of inflammatory substances.

Uses For relief from migraine, put one or two medium-sized, fresh leaves between two small slices of bread and eat them slowly when attacks are anticipated. Feverfew was traditionally used to treat fevers, to calm the nerves and to relieve painful periods and rheumatic pains, again reflecting its anti-inflammatory activity. You can also use a tincture or infusion of feverfew topically to relieve the pain and swelling of insect bites and as an insect repellent.

Dosage and preparations
Tincture – 1:5, 25%, or of the fresh herb 1:2, 45%, 1–2 ml.
Infusion – 1 g per cup, steeped for 5 minutes.
Fresh leaf – as above.
Many shop-bought feverfew tablets do not work very well; the fresh herb is best.

Cautions and contraindications
Feverfew should not be taken by children, or during pregnancy. It can cause mouth ulcers or stomach upsets in a small minority of people.

124

Taraxacum officinale DANDELION

Dandelion is a highly adaptable plant thought to originate in the foothills of central Asia, and is widely distributed throughout the Northern Hemisphere. The leaf and root are collected for medicinal purposes in spring. The root is also harvested in autumn when it is less bitter and higher in inulin, a kind of sugar. It is then roasted to make dandelion coffee.

The leaf and root contain vitamins A, C and D and the B vitamins. The leaf is especially rich in potassium and vitamin A and the root contains a large amount of starch. Both, but especially the root, contain a bitter latex – a milky kind of sap which becomes rubbery when dried. Indeed, a strain of dandelion was specially cultivated to augment the scarce and valuable supply of rubber needed to equip the Soviet Army in the Second World War. Young leaves are refreshing in salads and both root and leaf have proved valuable foods in times of famine.

Actions Dandelion is possibly the most widely prescribed medicinal plant in Western herbalism. It is used to improve the removal of fluid waste and stimulate liver function. The liver is extremely important and is involved in most of the intricate metabolic pathways of the body, and herbalists see healthy liver activity as vital to the harmonious functioning of the digestive and eliminative processes. Dandelion leaf is a potent diuretic, yet also replaces the potassium that is lost due to increased urine production, a common side effect of diuretics. It is also a bitter digestive stimulant that promotes bile excretion. The root is used as a liver tonic, digestive stimulant and a mild laxative.

Uses Dandelion is excellent for relieving all conditions where the digestion and metabolism are sluggish and as a cleansing herb for arthritis, gout and skin problems. The leaf, traditionally used in spring as a cleansing infusion, is used to treat water retention and rheumatism. The latex of the stalk can be used to remove warts by dabbing the wart every day over a number of weeks, taking care not to touch the surrounding skin.

Taraxacum officinale

Dosage and preparations
Tincture – 1:5, 25%, 1–2 ml.
Infusions and decoctions – 3–10 g leaf or root per cup, 3–4 times daily.
Fresh juice of leaf and root – 3–5 ml.

Cautions and contraindications
The flower stalks are not edible and the latex in them can cause a brown stain on the skin. Children should be warned against sucking them.

125

Thymus vulgaris THYME

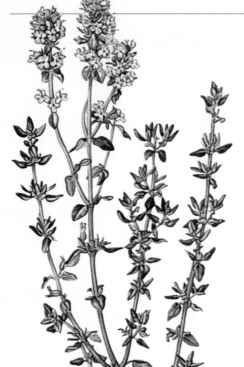

Thyme is native to the Mediterranean coast and likes well-drained, lime-rich soil. The flowering herb contains volatile oil, tannins, bitters, flavonoids and saponins. Thyme is often grown in gardens and is used in cooking. Wild thyme (*Thymus serpyllum*) has similar properties.

Actions Thyme is a useful expectorant and relaxes bronchial spasm (tightness of the airways) and improves fluid secretions. It is partly excreted via the lungs and is a very powerful antiseptic which gives it a useful range of actions – soothing a cough, liquefying mucus and acting as a disinfectant. Thyme essential oil is both antifungal and vermicidal (though non-toxic internally). As a digestive herb thyme helps to prevent infection and is an aromatic stimulant and carminative.

Uses Thyme is excellent for infectious or dry coughs, whooping cough and bronchitis. As an antiseptic herb it is a good mouthwash and gargle for sore gums, sore throats and laryngitis. It is also a useful lotion for thrush, athlete's foot and other fungal infections. As a digestive herb it is helpful for poor appetite and flatulence.

Dosage and preparations
Tincture – 1:5, 45%, 2–6 ml.
Infusion – 2–4 g per cup, steeped for 5–10 minutes.

Cautions and contraindications
Avoid taking during pregnancy. Thyme's essential oil should be well diluted to avoid irritation through topical use.

Thymus vulgaris

Tilia europea LIME

Lime trees are large and leafy, and commonly found throughout Europe. The flowers and the bracts (leafy structures around the base of the flowers), present from May to July, are rich in flavonoids, saponins, mucilage, tannins, sugars, and a tiny amount of a substance similar to chemical tranquillisers.

Actions Limeflower can be used as a sedative, a relaxant, an antispasmodic and a vasodilator (an agent that widens and relaxes blood vessels). It can also be used as a diaphoretic and has diuretic properties.

Uses With their mild, pleasant taste, limeflowers are among the most popular herbal relaxants. They are useful in treating anxiety, migraine and a range of circulatory problems, including palpitations and varicose veins. The saponins and flavonoids are thought to have a beneficial effect on the blood vessel walls in people with hardening of the arteries, and limeflower is one of the major herbs used to treat high blood pressure. As a diaphoretic, limeflower is good for feverish colds and catarrh, particularly in children.

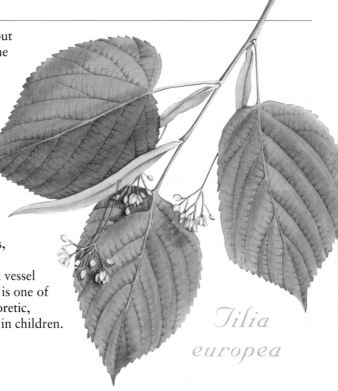

Tilia europea

Dosage and preparations
Tincture – 1:5, 25%, 1–2 ml.
Infusion – 2 teaspoons per cup infused for no more than 5 minutes.

Cautions and contraindications
Infusions made from old, stale leaves can reportedly cause sensations of drunkenness.

Trifolium pratense RED CLOVER

The flowerheads of this familiar meadow plant are reddish-purple and the leaves consist of three oval leaflets. It is common throughout Europe and in central and eastern Asia. The flowerheads contain flavonoids and a little volatile oil. Flavonoids in the leaves include several which act like the hormone oestrogen found naturally in the body.

Actions Though one of the most commonly used 'blood cleansing' herbs, red clover's medicinal actions have not been thoroughly researched. It is prescribed by herbalists as a dermatological agent and alterative, a mild antispasmodic and an expectorant.

Uses Used to treat psoriasis and eczema, both orally and externally. It is also a relaxing expectorant, helpful for coughs, bronchitis and whooping cough, and can be particularly beneficial for children suffering from both asthma and eczema. It is also used as a treatment for some cancers.

Trifolium pratense

Dosage and preparations
Tincture – 1:5, 25%, in alcohol or glycerol, 2–5 ml.
Infusion – 2–4 g per cup.
An ointment for psoriasis can be made by boiling down a concentrated decoction until it reaches a thick, tarry consistency.

Cautions and contraindications
A glycerol extract or infusion may be better for skin problems, avoiding the diaphoretic effect of alcohol.

Trigonella foenum-graecum FENUGREEK

Fenugreek is indigenous to the eastern Mediterranean; its seeds have been used since antiquity as a food and a medicine and feature in Chinese, Indian, Arabic and Western herbal medicine. The seeds contain mucilage, a volatile oil, a bitter principle, steroidal saponins and an alkaloid.

Actions Fenugreek seeds are a nutritive digestive tonic and, when moistened, are both demulcent and emollient. They have a long history of use as a galactogogue and also as a male hormonal tonic. Overall, fenugreek could be characterised as a strengthening herb that is also locally soothing.

Uses The seeds are useful for convalescent states, especially those involving poor digestion, and for painful bowel problems where the mucilage acts to soothe and lubricate and to give the stool bulk and softness. Powdered and soaked overnight in water, fenugreek seeds can form a soothing, anti-inflammatory poultice for rheumatic pains, skin irritations and abrasions. Dry fenugreek powder makes a good drawing poultice applied topically to boils. An infusion or tincture helps milk production in nursing mothers and is used in China to treat impotence in men and menopausal problems in women. Applied topically it has been used to treat hair loss.

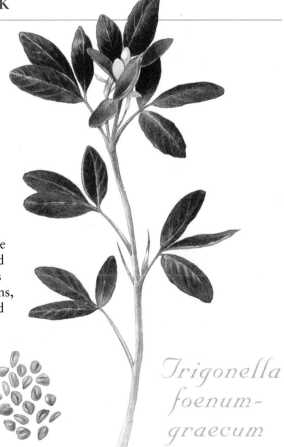

Trigonella foenum-graecum

Dosage and preparations
Tincture – 1:5, 45%, 2–4 ml.
Infusion – 2 g per cup infused for 5 minutes.
Powder – as poultice.

Cautions and contraindications
Avoid during pregnancy.

Tussilago farfara COLTSFOOT

Coltsfoot grows in boggy ground or heavy clay. The single, hairy stem, covered in leaf-scales, produces a bright yellow flower head in early spring. The leaves, to whose shape the name refers, reach full size in later spring. The leaves and flowers contain mucilage and the leaves also contain tannins.

Actions Coltsfoot is a relaxing expectorant that is soothing to bronchial irritation and liquefying to bronchial secretions. The leaves are rich in zinc and potassium nitrate, burn well and were the main ingredient of 'cigarettes' used by the Romans to treat asthma by inhaling the smoke through a reed. They are also vulnerary.

Uses A relaxing expectorant, useful for stubborn, tight coughs, for chronic chest problems and asthma. Coltsfoot is an excellent cough suppressant, especially for smokers and elderly people. The leaves can be used in a poultice or ointment for cuts and poorly healing wounds.

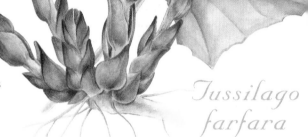

Tussilago farfara

Dosage and preparations
Tincture – 1:5, 25%, or fresh juice, 2–4 ml.
Infusion – 2–4 g per cup.
A syrup can be made from the fresh flowers.

Cautions and contraindications
Small amounts of pyrrolizidine alkaloids present in coltsfoot raise fears regarding its safety. Coltsfoot has been widely used for many centuries, with no record of ill effects, and the mucilage and tannins in the plant hinder the absorption of these alkaloids. Nevertheless, it would be wise to refrain from long-term internal use.

Urtica dioica NETTLE

Stinging nettle is a large perennial which likes cultivated, nitrogen-rich soil and makes an excellent organic fertiliser. It is harvested in May and June before flowering while the stinging hairs on the leaves and stalk are rich in histamine and serotonin. The whole herb contains flavonoids, vitamins and minerals, especially calcium and potassium salts and silicic acid.

Actions Nettles are excellent for regulating and optimising bodily functions and they are also a good cleansing and nutritive herb. Nettles cause increased elimination of sodium and urea, which is perhaps one reason why they have been found helpful in rheumatic and arthritic conditions because a build-up of these substances exacerbates these conditions. The fresh root is now widely prescribed for prostate hypertrophy (enlargement) and irritable bladders in older men.

Uses Nettles are helpful for skin problems and arthritis associated with poor circulation. They are also useful for allergic or irritable skin and respiratory problems, including asthma and urticaria (nettle rash). They have been used for centuries to promote milk production, both in humans and animals. A nettle infusion is a good spring cleansing tonic and a help in congestive conditions and water retention.

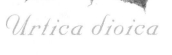

Urtica dioica

Dosage and preparations
Tincture – 1:5, 25%, 5 ml.
Infusion – 1–3 g per cup.
Fresh juice – 30 ml.

Cautions and contraindications
None known.

Vaccinium myrtillus BILBERRY

Bilberry grows in the hilly areas of northern Europe and the USA, where it is also known as huckleberry. In Europe it is sometimes called wild blueberry. Bilberry is a small, leathery-leaved shrub producing slightly acid-tasting berries containing tannins, vitamin C and minerals such as manganese, phosphorus, iron and zinc.

Actions Bilberry is astringent and antispasmodic with anti-inflammatory and mildly sedative properties. It is mildly antibacterial and the tannins probably account for its antidiarrhoeal action. Bilberry also has a frequently observed improvement in eyesight disorders, especially poor night vision. The active constituents strengthen the capillaries and veins, improve peripheral circulation and regulate the flow of blood.

Uses Only the berries are used. Bilberry is useful both as a treatment for diarrhoea and as a herb to aid circulation, with particular application for eye problems including cataracts, diabetic-induced glaucoma, poor night vision and eye strain. It is also used in association with circulatory or inflammatory conditions such as allergic reactions, hypertension or poor circulation and nerve and kidney problems resulting from fragile capillaries. Varicose veins are also relieved by bilberry.

Dosage and preparations
Tincture – 1:4, 25%, 5–10 ml.
Berries – fresh 2–4 g, dried 1 g.

Cautions and contraindications
None known.

Vaccinium myrtillus

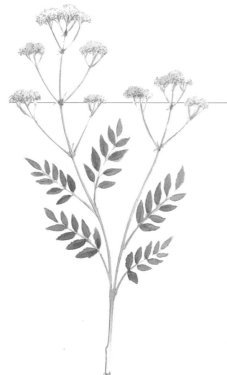

Valeriana officinalis VALERIAN

A perennial that grows up to 1 m (3 ft) in height. Species of valerian are found in all temperate regions of the world. The rhizomes, roots and stolons (runners) are harvested during the autumn and carefully dried at temperatures below 40°C. Valerian contains volatile oil and alkaloids. The combination of different constituents seems essential to its overall effects.

Actions The many studies of valerian's actions have established its mildly sedative, antispasmodic and pain-relieving effects. Taken an hour before retiring, valerian shortens the time taken to go to sleep and improves general sleep quality. It is also relaxing to the digestive system when it is affected by nervous tension.

Uses Valerian calms nervous tension and stress, useful for pre-examination nerves, nervous palpitations, skin problems that are exacerbated by anxiety or nervousness, nervous exhaustion and tension headaches. It is also highly useful in nervous digestive problems, such as occasional constipation and irritable bowel syndrome.

Valeriana officinalis

Dosage and preparations
Tincture – 1:5, 45 %, 2–4 ml.
Infusion – 2–5 g infused for 10 minutes.

Cautions and contraindications
Valerian is very safe even at high doses, but prolonged high doses can lead to irritability. A few people find valerian overstimulating or that it gives them headaches.

Verbascum thapsus MULLEIN

A tall biennial, common on dry roadsides and wasteland, mullein is densely covered with white woolly hairs. The name *Verbascum* is derived from the Latin, *barba*, meaning beard. The stem appears in the second year, bearing a long spike of yellow flowers. This used to be dipped in tar and used as a torch as the hairs were easily ignited. The leaves and flowers contain mucilage, saponins, flavonoids and traces of volatile oil.

Actions Mullein is expectorant, demulcent and a soothing diuretic.

Uses Excellent for coughs, especially tight, dry and irritable coughs, mullein is specifically indicated for hoarseness, whooping cough, wheezy asthma and bronchitis. The flowers are more strongly expectorant than the leaves, which are a soothing diuretic for irritation in the urinary tract. The infused oil, common in pharmacies as ear drops until recent times, is emollient and soothing and is used for earache and as a rub for inflamed joints. The bruised leaf is an old gardener's cure for haemorrhoids.

Dosage and preparations
Tincture – 1:5, 25%, 3–5 ml.
Infusion – 4–8 g of leaves or
1–4 g of flowers per cup.

Cautions and contraindications
Infusions should be carefully strained to filter out the fine hairs which can irritate the throat.

Verbascum thapsus

Verbena officinalis L. VERVAIN

A slender, erect perennial, bearing small white or lilac-coloured flowers in long slender spikes, vervain grows by roadsides and in sunny pastures. The aerial parts are harvested just at flowering when they contain the glycosides verbenin and verbenalin, a bitter principle, tannins and volatile oil.

Actions Thymoleptic and mildly sedative, androgenic (increasing male hormones), emmenagogue, galactogogue, astringent, insecticidal, diaphoretic, vervain is a gentle and versatile favourite with many herbalists. Country names include 'simpler's joy' (a simple is a herb used alone to treat problems) and 'traveller's joy'. In Germany it is known as 'Ironwort' (Eisenkraut) because of its use in treating wounds caused by iron weapons.

Uses Vervain is a calming restorative for debilitating conditions, particularly nervous exhaustion and depression. It is antiseptic to wounds and makes an excellent mouthwash for dental and gum disease. It relieves poor menstrual flow associated with coldness and poor milk flow. In traditional Chinese medicine it is used as a blood detoxifier and for throat swellings.

Dosage and preparations
Tincture – 1:5, 25%, up to 5 ml.
Infusions – 2–4 g per cup; can also be used as a lotion.

Cautions and contraindications
None known.

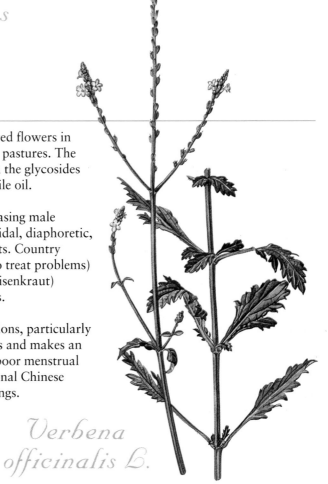

Verbena officinalis L.

Viburnum opulus CRAMP BARK
Viburnum prunifolium BLACK HAW

Cramp bark is the stem bark from the guelder rose shrub, a native of the USA and Europe which grows in woodlands. Similar in appearance to a small elder, the guelder rose has flat-topped clusters of white flowers, larger than elderflowers, and large bright red berries. The bark contains a bitter resin and tannins. Black haw is a shrub or small tree indigenous to the USA, which is characterised by its short, pointed winter buds and sharply pointed leaves. Black haw berries are bluish-black. The stem and root bark are used and contain tannins and saponins.

Actions Both species are antispasmodic, black haw more specifically for uterine spasm (menstrual cramping). Cramp bark is used as a muscle and nerve relaxant.

Uses Cramp bark is beneficial in all conditions where anxiety together with muscular tension or cramps feature, such as tension headaches, colic and asthma. A strong infusion is very effective applied as a lotion for muscle cramps and spasms. Black haw is used more for menstrual problems including threatened miscarriage, excessive menstrual bleeding and pain. Always seek professional herbal or medical advice before self-treatment.

Viburnum prunifolium

Viburnum opulus

Dosage and preparations
Tincture – 1:5, 25%, 3–8 ml. Infusion – 1–3 g of dried powder infused or simmered for 10 minutes.

Cautions and contraindications
Avoid cramp bark during pregnancy. Fresh cramp bark berries are poisonous.

Vitex agnus castus AGNUS CASTUS

Agnus castus is a Mediterranean shrub related to vervain, whose dried fruits have been used since antiquity to restrain sexual desire and nervous excitability. It contains a volatile oil, flavonoids and a bitter principle.

Actions Agnus castus berries shift the balance of hormones produced by the pituitary gland affecting the menstrual cycle. The overall effect of this is to increase the production of progesterone, leading to a reduction in premenstrual irritability, breast tenderness and water retention.

Uses Agnus castus is one of the main herbal hormone tonics with a wide range of applications. It helps to regulate the menstrual cycle, especially frequent or heavy bleeding, and premenstrual symptoms such as breast tenderness and irritability. It promotes lactation in nursing mothers, helps reduce acne where hormonally related, and encourages normal ovulation and menstruation. It can reduce menopausal complaints, such as hot flushes. For best results take agnus castus for long periods of time.

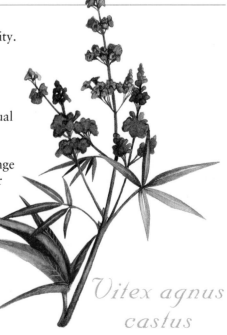

Vitex agnus castus

Dosage and preparations
Tincture – 1:5, 25%, 2–4 ml.
Powdered fruits – 0.3–1 g in the morning.

Cautions and contraindications
None known.

Zea mays CORNSILK

Cornsilk consists of the stigmas and styles (the silky strands emerging from the cob) of sweetcorn or maize. They contain insoluble sugars – mannitol, inositol and sorbitol – a large amount of potassium, flavonoids, silica and a small amount of volatile oil. Cornsilk should be used fresh for best effect.

Actions Cornsilk is a slightly demulcent soothing diuretic and a mild urinary antiseptic. Like dandelion leaf, it compensates for potassium lost through increased urine output by its high potassium content.

Uses An infusion taken several times a day soothes and calms the irritation of cystitis while helping to deal with the infection itself. It is not powerfully antiseptic and is best combined with antiseptic herbs like thyme and juniper. It is a useful herb in acute or chronic cystitis and its diuretic properties are helpful in treating water retention. Because of its soothing quality, it is also useful for relieving an irritable or nervous bladder and as such is particularly recommended for reducing bed-wetting in children.

Dosage and preparations
Tincture – 1:5, 25%, 2–4 ml.
Infusion – 2 g per cup.

Cautions and contraindications
None known.

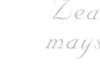

Zea mays

Zingiber officinalis GINGER

Ginger is Asian in origin but widely cultivated in the USA, the West Indies, India and Africa. The root is used both fresh and dried and contains varying proportions of volatile constituents depending on the area of origin and method of drying.

Actions A strong circulatory stimulant with anticlotting, anti-inflammatory and vasodilatory effects. When chewed, ginger temporarily increases blood pressure, but not when swallowed without chewing. It is a warming digestive stimulant and antispasmodic, an antiemetic, particularly when dried, and an antiseptic expectorant. The fresh root has a gentler, more peripheral action, while the dried root is a strong central stimulant with a more powerful digestive action, together with an ability to inhibit one of the most prevalent and widespread common cold viruses.

Uses Ginger is a reliable travel sickness remedy, it is helpful for poor digestion, especially accompanied by cold, and for colic, flatulence and diarrhoea. Ginger tea will help to sweat out a cold, is anticatarrhal, helpful for coughs and eases menstrual cramps accompanied by cold. It can also be of benefit for easing chronic inflammatory conditions such as arthritis (not during flare-ups, however), and helps cold hands and feet.

Dosage and preparations
Tincture – 1:5, 60%, 5–20 drops.
Ginger sweets are helpful for nausea and travel sickness.

Cautions and contraindications
Avoid during acute inflammation – ginger is too heating to give relief.

Zingiber officinalis

CHAPTER 6

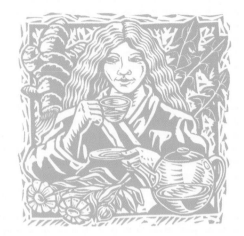

HEALING WITH HERBS

*Self-healing with herbs can be an effective,
simple and safe form of treatment for many
minor conditions. From nausea to gout, there
is a selection of herbal remedies that can be
applied to offer speedy relief from symptoms
and hinder or prevent recurrence. This chapter
reveals a range of home remedies, available to
all, which draw on the remarkable secrets
of herbal healing.*

DIGESTIVE SYSTEM PROBLEMS

Digestive disorders can range from uncomfortable indigestion to dangerous and painful inflammation such as colitis. Herbal preparations can help to relieve and prevent such problems.

When the body fails to digest food adequately, or reacts to foods or events, such as sea travel, with diarrhoea or nausea, the physical results can be highly discomforting and often painful. Conventional treatments can be aggressive and harsh on the digestive system: herbal remedies can often provide a gentler but equally effective alternative.

NAUSEA, VOMITING AND MOTION SICKNESS

Nausea may be a sign of liver disease or nervous tension, and often occurs in the early stages of pregnancy. In all these cases, the underlying cause of the condition should be diagnosed by a doctor and, where necessary, treated medically.

For other bouts of nausea where you are sure the problem is short-lived, such as travel sickness, ginger root can be used. Fresh ginger root is the traditional remedy for nausea and vomiting in both Ayurvedic and Tibetan medicine and modern studies and clinical trials have confirmed its ancient uses. For acute nausea a fresh piece of the root chewed slowly is very effective or alternatively it may be drunk as a hot infusion. Ginger is a hot spice and people with a sensitive stomach might not tolerate it.

Motion sickness is triggered by sudden movements, like a ship rocking, and causes nausea, vomiting and dizziness. Black horehound has strong antiemetic properties, although clinical trials to prove its effectiveness have not been conclusive. It has an unpleasant taste and is easier to take as a tincture in small doses – 5 drops every hour for acute nausea – rather than as a tea.

LOSS OF APPETITE AND WEAK DIGESTION

Although some people naturally have a weak digestion, an inexplicable loss of appetite may be a symptom of liver disease, of an emotional problem such as depression

HERBS AND THE DIGESTIVE SYSTEM

Many herbs act on the digestive system, either to soothe or stimulate, and herbal remedies can help to relieve many digestive disorders, from vomiting to wind.

Before you begin treatment make sure you clearly understand your symptoms – some digestive disorders can indicate more serious underlying problems.

Gentian, mugwort and centaury are recommended for loss of appetite

Meadowsweet and marshmallow are stomachic herbs that will relieve acid indigestion

Liquorice contains mucilage that helps to relieve the pain of stomach ulcers

Ginger and black horehound have antiemetic actions that help to relieve nausea

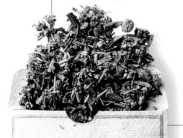

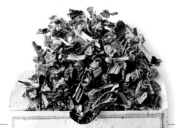

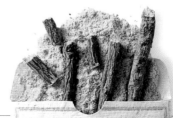

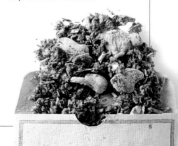

or your body's response to an acute illness. You should consult your doctor if you lose your appetite for more than two days.

Gentian and mugwort both belong to the group of bitter remedies which stimulate the appetite and improve digestion. They are good remedies to restore digestive function during convalescence. Due to their extremely bitter taste they are best taken as tinctures in small doses; 5–10 drops before meals until your appetite returns to normal.

Centaury is a bitter and astringent tonic which stimulates the appetite and strengthens the digestive tract in general. It has been shown to be effective where there is a general weakness of the digestive system. It is gentle enough to be given to children either as a tea – ¼ teaspoon centaury in ½ cup boiling water to be taken before meals – or as a tincture – only for children over 5 years, 5–10 drops to be taken in a little fruit juice two to three times a day before meals.

Adults should take 10–20 drops of centaury three times a day before meals. Its full benefits will be felt after two to three months of treatment. It is important that children under 5 years who suffer a diminished appetite should receive professional medical attention.

ACIDITY OF THE STOMACH AND ULCERS

Too much acid in the stomach can produce symptoms like heartburn and regurgitation of food after meals. It may also contribute to ulcers forming in the stomach or small intestine. Symptoms of ulcers include pain, indigestion and regurgitation; they are common, but can become very serious, so if you suspect an ulcer consult your doctor immediately. A bad diet and high stress levels can exacerbate ulcer problems.

Excess stomach acid should be treated with stomachic and demulcent herbs, like meadowsweet and marshmallow, which

Holiday Herbal First Aid

Many holidaymakers find that the sudden change in diet, alcohol intake and water quality during their holiday causes stomach disorders. These can range from mild indigestion to serious bouts of diarrhoea and constipation. If a stomach upset is caused by an infection, herbal remedies can relieve the symptoms, but the infection must be treated too. Otherwise, a simple herbal first aid kit designed to focus on the digestive system can help to prevent and relieve the various problems caused by holiday stomach upsets.

help to regulate the acid content of the stomach. For best effects they should be taken as tinctures over long periods of time. Mix meadowsweet and marshmallow tinctures equally and take 1 teaspoon of the mixture in a little water three times a day before meals. Dietary changes should include cutting out fatty and fried foods as well as rich, heavy meals. Coffee and alcohol should also be avoided.

Liquorice has been shown to be an effective aid in the treatment of ulcers and recent research has confirmed the use of the root as a demulcent and anti-inflammatory remedy. The fresh root yields a thick, sweet juice which should be diluted with hot water and drunk as a tea. It may also be taken as a tincture – 1 teaspoon tincture in a little water three times a day – but long-term use should be carefully monitored because liquorice can cause water retention and raise blood pressure. Liquorice should not be used by people who suffer from high blood pressure.

CONSTIPATION

This is a very common condition and is often caused by a low-fibre diet and lack of exercise. Stressful situations and liver disorders may also contribute, although some people are simply prone to a lazy bowel so constipation may become chronic.

Psyllium (plantain) seeds are a type of bulk-producing laxative. Taken internally they soak up water as they pass through the digestive tract, expanding in volume as they do so. Their bulk stimulates the bowel wall to cause a bowel motion. Psyllium seeds are indigestible and can produce wind, and so are best taken with carminative herbs like fennel or angelica. Sprinkle 1–2 teaspoons of psyllium seeds with a pinch of

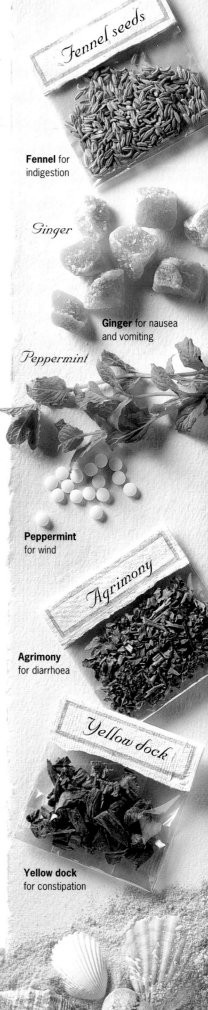

Fennel for indigestion

Ginger for nausea and vomiting

Peppermint for wind

Agrimony for diarrhoea

Yellow dock for constipation

Constipation

Constipation is one of the most common health problems in the Western world. Although not a disease in itself, constipation can be a symptom of an underlying condition or may be caused by an inappropriate diet, lack of exercise or nervous tension.

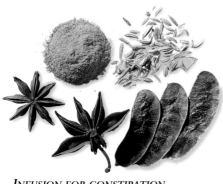

INFUSION FOR CONSTIPATION
Treat occasional constipation with rhubarb powder, a pinch of powdered fennel, senna pods or star anise.

Some people naturally have a lazy bowel and either have difficulty in passing stools or suffer infrequent bowel movements. This form of chronic constipation may be a sign of underlying liver problems.

In all cases of constipation it is important that the cause be identified and treated, although herbal remedies and simple dietary changes can help to relieve constipation and keep your digestion healthy.

CONSTIPATION BEATERS

It is well established that a low-fibre diet is a major cause of constipation. Fibre is the indigestible part of the food we eat and is found in large amounts in cereals (wheat, rye, oats and barley), pulses (beans, chickpeas and lentils), seeds (linseed, sesame, pumpkin) and fruit and vegetables. Dietary fibre makes up the bulk of stools and stimulates peristalsis, the rhythmic contraction of the bowel walls that moves food through the gut. The more fibre you eat, the more frequent, easy and complete your bowel movements will become, but you must also increase your fluid intake to soften stools.

Drink at least 2–4 pints (1–2 litres) of fluid every day. Mineral or filtered water is best.

Herbal laxatives
Occasional constipation may be treated with stimulant laxatives, such as Chinese rhubarb and senna. Take them as a syrup or tincture before going to bed to produce a bowel movement the following morning. If constipation lasts for more then three days, seek medical advice. All stimulant laxatives should be avoided during pregnancy and by sufferers of inflammatory bowel disease or those who are very weak.

Herbal bulking agents
Plant seeds like psyllium or linseed contain large amounts of mucilage and cellulose which can expand up to three times in volume as they pass through the gut. By doing so they help to make stools larger, softer and smoother. When you take bulking agents make sure you drink at least one glass of liquid at the same time to ensure they work properly. Taken in this way they will produce a bowel motion after 6–12 hours.

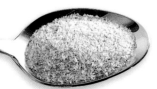

BREAKFAST BOOST
Sprinkle 1–2 teaspoons of psyllium or linseed seeds on yoghurt or muesli every day. Add a pinch of ground fennel to counteract flatulence.

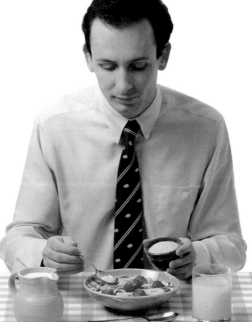

FIBRE IN YOUR DIET

At least two-thirds of your daily meals should be high in fibre:

▶ *Cereals – porridge oats, muesli and brown rice.*
▶ *Pulses – red and green lentils and beans.*
▶ *Seeds – sesame, sunflower, pumpkin and linseed.*
▶ *Fruits – apples, oranges, apricots and pears.*
▶ *Vegetables – celery, carrots, pumpkin and brussels sprouts.*

ground fennel on muesli or yoghurt and eat this with a cup of herbal tea each evening until the constipation passes.

Stimulant laxatives work by irritating the bowel wall, causing it to contract and expel its contents. Senna, Chinese rhubarb and aloe belong to this group. Stimulant laxatives can be taken as tinctures, but are more effective and kinder to the digestive tract if taken in syrup form: 1–2 teaspoons taken before going to bed will produce a bowel movement in the morning. It is best to combine stimulant laxatives with carminative herbs like fennel or angelica.

DIARRHOEA AND COLITIS

Diarrhoea can be a sign of an acute infection, or the result of a stressful situation or over-excitement. Treatment for diarrhoea uses gentle astringent herbs to reduce the amount of fluid lost.

Agrimony is a mild but effective remedy which is especially suitable for diarrhoea in children. Other suitable herbs include meadowsweet and lady's mantle. These are best taken as a tea, to replace lost fluids, 1 cup four times a day. Continue treatment until symptoms pass – if they last for more than two days, consult your doctor.

Colitis affects the large intestine where the bowel wall becomes inflamed. It causes alternating diarrhoea and constipation and can be very painful. Colitis should always be treated by a doctor.

To relieve the symptoms of colitis, agrimony combines well with meadowsweet to make an effective tea; take 1 cup, four times a day. Marigold may be added for its anti-inflammatory effect. Studies have shown that agrimony is particularly effective for chronic conditions such as inflammation of the bowel, but the remedies must be taken for at least two to three months.

CAUTION
Stimulant laxatives may cause griping pains and should never be taken by pregnant women, people with an inflammatory disease of the bowel (colitis) or those who are very weak. If you are unsure about stimulant laxatives, seek advice from a professional herbalist before self-treatment.

Leaves for Digestion

A good way to boost a flagging or weakened digestive system is to increase the herbs in your diet. Herbs with a bitter action promote the production of the stomach's juices which serve to break down food. Other herbs have a calming effect and help to settle the stomach after eating. Indigestion can be relieved with carminative herbs. Use fresh herbs liberally in salads. Alternatively, you can steam or wilt them in a little hot water and serve them as vegetables.

LIVER AND GALL BLADDER PROBLEMS

Symptoms of liver and gall bladder disease include indigestion, nausea, headaches, constipation, jaundice and excessive burping, all of which are very common. Often a bad diet rich in fatty foods, excessive alcohol intake and a generally unhealthy lifestyle can contribute. Both organs can develop serious problems, such as hepatitis or gallstones, so medical advice should be sought if you have any concerns about the seriousness of your condition.

Dandelion, milk thistle and mugwort are herbs that gently stimulate the liver and gall bladder to produce and secrete enough bile to ensure a healthy digestion. These herbs can be found in many old herbal cures and recent clinical studies have confirmed their claims for therapeutic actions. Dry roasted dandelion root makes a pleasant drink and should be prepared as a decoction. Drink 1 cup each day as a substitute for coffee.

Milk thistle and mugwort are best taken as tinctures – 1 teaspoon two to three times a day with a little water. Mugwort should be avoided during pregnancy.

INDIGESTION AND COLIC

The discomfort that occurs after overeating, eating too quickly or eating the wrong foods is described as indigestion and can be very painful. Herbs like fennel, angelica and peppermint dispel wind and thus relieve the discomfort of indigestion. For best results, take these herbs as a hot tea; sip 1 cup slowly after meals.

Colic pains are due to intense muscle spasms in the gut and can be caused by wind or nervous tension. Peppermint is particularly effective for colic pains because of its strongly antispasmodic action. It should be combined with camomile in a tea, 1 cup taken after each meal.

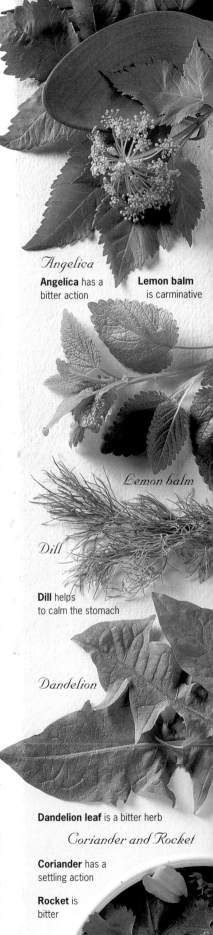

Angelica

Angelica has a bitter action

Lemon balm is carminative

Lemon balm

Dill

Dill helps to calm the stomach

Dandelion

Dandelion leaf is a bitter herb

Coriander and Rocket

Coriander has a settling action

Rocket is bitter

RESPIRATORY PROBLEMS

Disorders that restrict breathing, whether affecting the nose, lungs or airways, can cause serious discomfort. Many herbal remedies can help to relieve and clear congestion.

Commonly caused by either allergic reactions, viruses and infections, respiratory problems can be chronic or acute. In addition to the discomfort of laboured breathing, coughing and wheezing can cause muscular pain, headaches and dizziness. Herbal remedies act to soothe inflamed membranes, clear blocked airways and relax constricted muscles. Any persistent or worsening respiratory disorder should be treated by a doctor.

ASTHMA

Characterised by a tight chest, wheezing and coughing, asthma is the result of a constriction of the airways. A severe asthma attack can be very serious and should be treated by a doctor. The condition may be hereditary or due to an allergic reaction to dust, pollen or animal fur.

Modern and traditional herbalists use the Chinese herb Ma Huang to treat asthma. Ma Huang has a powerful action which dilates the airways and reduces the bronchial spasms that are characteristic of an asthma attack. It is not commonly available and can only be prescribed by a qualified professional herbalist. Ma Huang has a mild hypertensive action and should not be taken by people with high blood pressure.

Demulcent and antitussive herbs such as marshmallow, mullein and coltsfoot help soothe the irritated airways and keep them working. Camomile is particularly useful for childhood asthma if the condition is linked to nervous tension. All these herbs can be taken as tinctures, 1 teaspoon three times a day; teas, 3 cups a day; or syrups, 2 teaspoons three times a day, and should be used over long periods of time. Children over 5 years old should take half the adult dose. Do not give to younger children.

BRONCHITIS

An infection of the lower airways, bronchitis usually results in wheezing and coughing up yellow or green phlegm. It may also be accompanied by a fever.

The herbal treatment of bronchitis concentrates on antitussive and expectorant remedies. Thyme, coltsfoot and mullein leaf soothe the inflamed bronchi and calm excessive coughing. Expectorant herbs like hyssop and elecampane make a cough more productive – expressing more phlegm – and free the airways. The herbs should be taken as syrups or tinctures as short term remedies – take either 1 teaspoon tincture or 2 teaspoons syrup every four hours. Seek medical advice if attacks last more than four days.

HAY FEVER

Hay fever, or allergic rhinitis, is an abnormal immune response to flowers, grass or tree pollen and is particularly severe during the summer months. Symptoms include

THYME AND EUCALYPTUS INHALANT Steam inhalations made from thyme and eucalyptus can help to keep the airways clear. Using these herbs as inhalants delivers their antiseptic properties straight to the bronchi. Add 10 drops of thyme and eucalyptus essential oils to a bowl of hot water and breathe the steam two or three times daily during acute attacks of bronchitis.

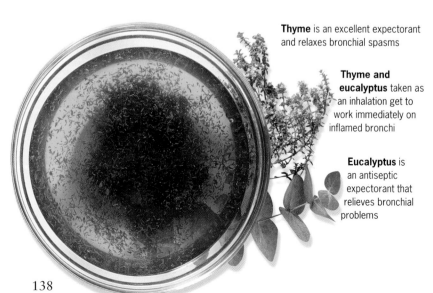

Thyme is an excellent expectorant and relaxes bronchial spasms

Thyme and eucalyptus taken as an inhalation get to work immediately on inflamed bronchi

Eucalyptus is an antiseptic expectorant that relieves bronchial problems

THYME AND COLTSFOOT SYRUP

Thyme and coltsfoot syrup is a very good base to which other herbs may be added as needed. Depending on the nature of your cough you may wish to include other herbs to tailor your remedy specifically. Demulcent and expectorant herbs will help to relieve a rattling, irritating cough.

Ingredients
1 litre (1¾ pints) filtered water
55 g (2 oz) dried thyme
55 g (2 oz) dried coltsfoot leaves
 or flowers
450 g (1 lb) castor sugar

1 *Bring the water to the boil in a stainless steel saucepan, stir in the dried herbs and simmer gently over a medium heat for 10 minutes.*

2 *Strain the decoction through a muslin cloth or clean tea towel, taking care to squeeze out the residue. Be careful: the herbs may be hot.*

3 *Transfer the liquid to a china bowl and place over a small saucepan one-third full of water.*

4 *Bring the water to the boil and let the decoction reduce slowly down to 250 ml (9 fl oz). This will take approximately 1–2 hours.*

5 *Remove the bowl from the saucepan and add the sugar. Stir the mixture continuously until the sugar has completely dissolved, then leave to cool. When cool pour into a dark bottle, label and store in a cool place.*

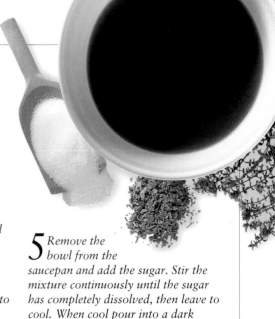

sneezing, a runny nose, itchy, swollen eyes and breathing difficulties, and can last from spring to early autumn.

Elderflower, plantain and eyebright have a tonic effect on the lining of the nose and throat and help them to resist seasonal attacks from pollen. Hay fever remedies should be taken either as teas or tinctures in standard doses (see page 85) over long periods of time. For best effects they must be taken throughout the year, not just at danger times or during attacks.

Chinese herbalists use the herb Ma Huang to treat acute attacks of hay fever because of its antiallergic properties. Nettle also has antiallergic properties and may safely be used instead of Ma Huang, which is not commonly available. Drink 1 cup of nettle tea up to four times a day.

COMMON COLD AND INFLUENZA
The common cold is a viral infection of the upper airways. Symptoms usually include sneezing, a runny nose with a yellow discharge, general malaise and sometimes fever. Influenza is an acute viral infection which causes a fever and muscle pain as well as coughing and a sore throat.

At the first sign of a cold or the flu take echinacea tincture or plenty of fresh garlic to give your immune system a boost. Both herbs are particularly good at fighting infections in the early stages. Take 2–5 ml of echinacea up to four times daily for about a week. There is no limit on your intake of garlic, except that imposed by taste.

An infusion made from peppermint, elderflower, yarrow and ginger will ease the worst symptoms of a cold and relieve the aches and pains of flu. It has warming and diaphoretic qualities and you should sip 3–4 cups a day while hot.

A hot bath with essential oils will also help to sweat out a cold, but should not be used in feverish conditions. Add a few drops of rosemary, eucalyptus or peppermint essential oils to a hot bath.

COUGH
A cough is the body's attempt to clear the lungs and bronchi of irritants or excess mucus. It can be a sign of an infection, such as bronchitis, or it may be a symptom of hay fever or nervous tension.

For a rattling cough use expectorant herbs to help the airways expel excess phlegm. Choose herbs that also have demulcent properties to soothe any irritation. Good expectorant herbs are mullein, elecampane, coltsfoot, angelica and hyssop. Mullein and coltsfoot combined have both demulcent and expectorant properties. Cough medicines are best taken as syrups as they soothe the inflamed airways and are easy to make at home (see above).

To relax the airways choose thyme or hyssop and for a chesty cough add expectorant herbs such as elecampane. Add 20 ml (⅔ fl oz)of tincture to 100 ml (3½ fl oz) of syrup base. Adults can take 10 ml (2 teaspoons) 3–4 times a day; children should take 5 ml (1 teaspoon) 3–4 times a day.

REPRODUCTIVE AND URINARY PROBLEMS

Some people find reproductive and urinary disorders distressing and embarrassing. Herbal remedies can help to relieve symptoms and reduce the frequency of urogenital problems.

*HERBS AND
MENSTRUAL PROBLEMS
For very heavy periods,
lady's mantle and
shepherd's purse help to
reduce excess bleeding.
They may be taken as a
tea or tincture, on their
own or in combination.
Cramping pains may
occur before a period
starts or during the first
two days. Cramp bark
tincture can be taken to
reduce cramping pains.
Take up to 3 teaspoons
in warm water three
times a day for acute
pains. Hot camomile tea
sipped slowly throughout
the day also soothes
period pains and relieves
diarrhoea.*

The majority of herbal remedies that offer relief from reproductive and urinary problems are taken internally as teas or tinctures, but some, such as those with antifungal properties, can be applied topically in ointments and creams.

PREMENSTRUAL SYNDROME (PMS)

Hormonal changes in the days leading up to a period can cause depression, irritability, anxiety, tenderness of the breasts and water retention. The severity and occurrence of these symptoms varies between individuals.

The most highly favoured herb for premenstrual syndrome is *Vitex agnus castus*. It has long been used to treat gynaecological problems and British studies have found that it is particularly effective at relieving the physical symptoms of PMS, such as water retention and tender breasts. To achieve the best results, take 20 drops of agnus castus tincture every morning for at least six months.

For emotional symptoms use gentle relaxing herbs such as camomile and lemon balm as teas throughout the month. Drink 1–2 cups daily, and 3–4 cups in the days leading up to your period.

MENOPAUSAL PROBLEMS

For months or even years before the menopause – the end of menstruation – a woman may experience both physical and emotional changes due to hormonal changes in the body. Research has recently been conducted into the hormone-regulating properties of *Rheum rhaponticum*, a species of rhubarb which is cultivated in Europe and America. The root of the plant is thought to have an oestrogenic action. Clinical discussions focus on the possible use of *Rheum rhaponticum* as a natural hormone replacement therapy. However, studies have not yet been conclusive and further research is being carried out.

Agnus castus can help to regulate menopausal hormonal changes. Sage tea that has been left to go cold is particularly effective taken against night sweats. Take 1 cup each night before bedtime. To ease stress, a standard dose (see page 84) of motherwort and lemon balm infusion should be taken each day.

SEXUAL IMPOTENCE

Impotence may be due to stress and nervous tension or caused by a physical problem such as prostatitis (inflammation of the prostate gland). Certain conventional drugs have also been found to reduce a man's ability to achieve or sustain an erection.

Some herbal tonics do have a specific action on the male reproductive system, like damiana and saw palmetto. Others have an

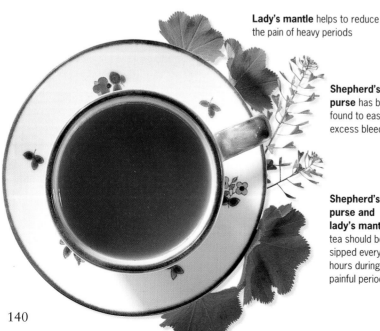

Lady's mantle helps to reduce the pain of heavy periods

Shepherd's purse has been found to ease excess bleeding

Shepherd's purse and lady's mantle tea should be sipped every few hours during painful periods

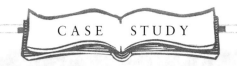
Painful Period Sufferer

Most women suffer from period pains at some time in their lives and although the causes are numerous they often include stress, bad eating habits and a lack of exercise. For many the pain is bearable, perhaps only mildly uncomfortable, but others suffer greatly. Fortunately, many menstrual problems respond very well to natural herbal remedies.

Julie is 26, single, and a landscape gardener. She greatly enjoys her job and is a lively and outgoing person with an active social life. Unfortunately, the pace of her life means she sometimes misses meals. For years Julie has had period problems – they tend to be very heavy with painful abdominal cramps two days before bleeding. She usually copes, but has had to take time off work because the pain is so bad. It can be eased with over-the-counter painkillers, but they do not relieve the nausea she often feels. Adding to her frustration, Julie has never had a regular menstrual cycle. Her doctor recommended she take oral contraceptives to regulate the periods and help to ease the pain, but Julie is reluctant to do so.

WHAT JULIE SHOULD DO

Julie has had painful periods for so long they are likely to be caused by hormonal imbalance. To regulate her hormone levels, Julie can take between 15–20 drops of agnus castus tincture every morning before breakfast. Agnus castus is a slow-acting remedy and should be taken for at least six months before definite improvements will show.

Julie should also take herbal tonics to improve the general health of her womb and ovaries. Herbs like marigold and lady's mantle are good tonics and can be taken as tinctures.

One to two cups of a hot, strong infusion of ginger and camomile taken four times a day in the days leading up to her period will ease Julie's cramps and nausea.

Action Plan

DIET
Increase intake of cold-pressed salad oils and oily fish as well as green leafy vegetables. Sesame seeds also contain a lot of calcium – calcium deficiency can exacerbate cramping.

LIFESTYLE
Take time to relax and unwind. Find a meditation class or go for long walks to release tension.

HEALTH
Herbal treatments can help to relieve all the symptoms of painful periods, as well as aiding relaxation.

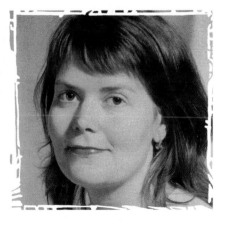

DIET
A lack of regular nutrition-rich foods can cause the body to respond badly to pain and extend recovery time.

LIFESTYLE
A hectic and busy life can cause tension which may exacerbate period pains. Anxiety and tiredness increase pain response.

HEALTH
Constant use of painkillers can increase fatigue and may cause side effects, such as nausea.

HOW THINGS TURNED OUT FOR JULIE

After four months of herbal treatment, Julie's periods are less painful but she still has cramps on the day before her period starts. She finds that the herbal tea stops the nausea and takes away the worst of the pain. Her menstrual cycle is still irregular, but she has noticed sufficient signs of a slow improvement to make her determined to continue the treatment, maintain her dietary improvements and learn more about stress-reduction.

indirect action, strengthening the body as a whole, like ginseng and other nerve tonics such as oats and skullcap. Research is looking at ginkgo's circulatory action, particularly in relation to the reproductive organs. All the herbs must be taken long-term as teas or tinctures in standard doses.

INFERTILITY

Infertility can be due to a number of causes and the majority of problems usually require long-term treatment. Any treatment should be carried out under professional supervision. Infertility that is caused by a hormone imbalance may respond well to *vitex agnus castus* taken daily every morning for at least six months.

Herbs that help keep the female reproductive system healthy include marigold, lady's mantle and raspberry. Marigold is beneficial for any underlying chronic inflammation of the reproductive system. Lady's mantle and raspberry are traditional tonic herbs for women which strengthen the womb and ovaries. All of these herbs can be taken every day as a tincture or as a tea.

THRUSH

A fungal infection caused by *Candida albicans*, thrush·most commonly affects the vagina causing irritation with itchy, red skin and a white, cloudy discharge. To treat thrush, use immune-stimulating herbs like echinacea, marigold and garlic. These are best taken in tincture form; 1 teaspoon up to four times a day for acute attacks. In addition, cleavers and marigold tea can be taken long-term to improve lymphatic drainage and thus help the immune system deal with the infection.

Combine internal treatment with external applications of antifungal herbs. Tea tree and thyme essential oils have been found to have particularly strong antifungal properties. Add 15–20 drops of each to 25 g (1 fl oz) base cream and apply twice daily for as long as symptoms persist. Infused oil of marigold reduces redness and irritation. A low-sugar diet will also help to fight thrush.

CYSTITIS

A common condition that affects mostly women, the symptoms of cystitis include an urgency to pass water, burning pain on urination and sometimes blood in the urine.

Herbs like juniper, plantain and yarrow are traditional remedies for urinary infections. They have a mild antiseptic action on the bladder and should be combined with demulcent herbs such as marshmallow and diuretics like dandelion leaf which will help to reduce the pain.

Take cystitis remedies as a tea – 1 cup every four hours – to help to flush out the bladder. Make sure you continue the course of treatment until all symptoms have disappeared. Use juniper with caution. It has a strong irritant action on the kidneys and should not be used by people with a kidney condition or during pregnancy.

PROSTATE ENLARGEMENT

A common condition in men over 40 years of age, enlargement of the prostate develops slowly and is characterised by an increasing difficulty and need to pass water. These symptoms should be checked by a doctor to exclude cancer of the prostate.

Saw palmetto, nettle and horsetail are recommended in traditional and modern herbal medicine for an enlarged prostate. Nettle root has been shown to be particularly beneficial in the early stages of prostate problems. For best results, nettle root should be taken as a tincture or prepared as a decoction, both taken in standard doses for long-term use (see page 84).

Herbal Myths

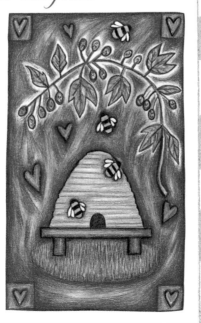

Hops that have been infused in boiling water, strained and mixed with honey make a simple modern equivalent of an ancient Teutonic female aphrodisiac. Known as honey-beer, new brides of ancient times would drink a mixture of fermented hops and honey each day for 30 days after their wedding ceremony to heighten their sexual responsiveness and increase their pleasure. This custom led to the term honeymoon being coined – 'moon' is an archaic and poetic term for a month.

HAIR AND SKIN PROBLEMS

From acne to dandruff, many health problems affect your skin and hair. The majority can be relieved and treated with readily available, simple and effective herbal remedies.

As the outside protective layer of the body, the skin is particularly susceptible to injury and infection. It is also true, however, that healthy skin and hair reflects the overall health of the body and is a useful diagnostic tool for doctors.

BRUISING
A blow to the skin can damage the capillaries beneath the surface, causing discoloration as blood spreads into the tissues. The discoloration varies between blue, green, brown, purple and yellow as the bruise heals. Most bruises are tender to the touch and are accompanied by swelling.

Prompt treatment can minimise swelling and discoloration. The astringent properties of witch hazel are well documented and a witch hazel compress is an excellent first aid treatment for a bruise. If bruising is accompanied by swelling and the skin feels very hot, a compress soaked in two parts witch hazel and one part cider vinegar will help. Compresses should cover the whole affected area and be changed frequently.

BURNS
Superficial burns with reddened skin and slight blistering may be treated at home. More serious and extensive burns must receive prompt professional medical attention. Burns should be treated straightaway with cool running water until the skin has cooled to normal temperature, then a few drops of lavender essential oil can be applied directly to the burn. This will help to keep the skin clean, reduce the pain and speed the healing process. Once the immediate trauma is over, anti-inflammatory herbs like marigold and St John's wort will help the burn to heal speedily. They may be used as creams or infused oils, applied liberally three or four times a day. Aloe vera gel may also help – it is very cooling and has anti-inflammatory properties.

CUTS AND GRAZES
Small cuts and grazes are easily treated at home, but deep wounds should be checked by a doctor to prevent infection.

A number of herbs are used to treat superficial wounds. Diluted marigold tincture has known antiseptic and anti-inflammatory properties and is useful to clean a dirty cut

MAKING A HERBAL SKIN SPRAY

Some skin conditions may be too painful to touch, which can make applying remedies a difficult and painful ordeal. A skin spray can apply herbal remedies directly to the skin without exacerbating problems and can soothe and cool painful skin disorders such as sunburn.

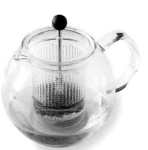

3 *Spray a light film of the preparation over the affected area and allow to evaporate.*

1 *Make an infusion or decoction of cooling or anti-inflammatory herbs such as marigold, lavender or camomile and lime flowers.*

2 *Pour the cooled liquid into a clean spray bottle, available from chemists, and secure the lid.*

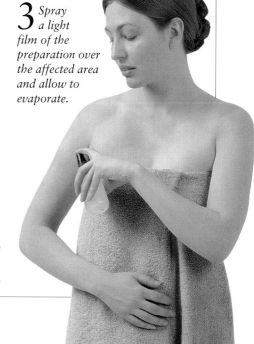

to prevent it from becoming infected. Echinacea tincture may be used in the same way. Dilute one part of tincture with three parts of water and use a sterile dressing pad to clean the cut and surrounding skin.

Inflamed and slow-healing wounds should be treated with comfrey, marigold or camomile ointment. Numerous studies have examined and confirmed the use of these herbs as wound healing remedies. Comfrey in particular is effective on slow-healing cuts and grazes and is known to prevent scar formation. Use in ointment form until the skin has healed completely.

WARTS, CORNS AND CALLUSES

Warts are viral infections of the skin which cause small, hard and uneven lesions, often on the hands and feet. Traditionally, the fresh juice of dandelion flower stalks was used to treat warts. It was applied directly over the wart to seal it until it disappeared. Slices of fresh garlic are also a reliable remedy. Apply for several minutes once a day until the wart has disappeared.

Corns and calluses are usually caused by ill-fitting shoes which put pressure on the skin of the foot, especially around the toes. The skin grows very thick and repeated friction may make the area inflamed and sore.

A cream with infused oil of marigold and essential oil of camomile can help to soothe red and inflamed feet. Massage the cream into your feet daily. Both herbs have excellent anti-inflammatory and wound-healing properties. For very thick corns, massage marigold oil ointment well into the skin every day. Ointments keep the skin soft and are good for use on small patches.

ATHLETE'S FOOT

Athlete's foot is a common fungal infection of the feet. The microbes that cause fungal infections thrive in warm, sweaty conditions such as those common in closed shoes, boots and trainers, and poor hygiene makes the problem worse. The condition is notoriously difficult to treat and requires both internal and external remedies.

Two to three cups of cleavers or marigold tea taken daily will help to improve lymphatic drainage and rid the body of fungal infections. Increased fresh garlic in the diet is also beneficial.

Externally, antifungal herbs like garlic, goldenseal, marigold and essential oil of tea tree or thyme should be applied daily. The tinctures can be used neat on the skin or mixed into a base cream. Scrupulous hygiene is also essential and feet must be dried thoroughly after washing and before treatments are applied. Although golden seal must not be used internally by pregnant women, it is completely safe to use externally in combination with other herbs.

PSORIASIS

Psoriasis occurs when skin cells overproduce causing patches of red, scaly itchy skin. The exact causes are unknown but attacks can be triggered by stress, and susceptibility to psoriasis often runs in families. Psoriasis is very common and can be severe.

The internal treatment of psoriasis is very similar to that of eczema (see below) using alterative and nervine herbs as appropriate. Evening primrose oil taken internally as capsules often helps to improve the elasticity of the skin and reduce the extent of dry and flaky skin patches.

Externally, herbal preparations should be rich and oily to moisturise the skin and reduce flakiness. Small patches of psoriasis can be treated with marigold, chickweed and marshmallow ointment to protect and soothe the skin. For large areas of psoriasis use infused oils of marigold, chickweed or even plain olive oil. Add peppermint if the skin is very itchy.

ECZEMA

The symptoms of eczema are red and sore patches on the skin, often in the crook of the elbow, behind the knees or on the hands. The affected skin can also become wet, weepy and extremely itchy. Some forms of

SORE FEET
Prolonged exercise and ill-fitting shoes are common causes of sore feet. The skin can develop painful blisters, which may burst and even bleed. Essential oil of peppermint is well known for its cooling action on the skin. Alternatively, make a strong infusion of peppermint, let it cool and use as a foot bath in the same way. Then massage your feet gently with marigold and camomile cream, taking care not to burst any blisters.

Peppermint foot cream

Mint footbath and peppermint cream can quickly relieve the pain of sore feet. Add 5 drops of peppermint oil to a bowl of cold water and bathe your feet in it for 10 minutes. This will cool and refresh tired, sore feet

Mint

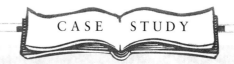

The Psoriasis Sufferer

Psoriasis is one of the most common skin diseases in the Western world, affecting up to 2 per cent of people. It is characterised by patches of red, itchy and scaly skin, and despite intensive research it remains difficult to treat. However, herbs and dietary changes can help to relieve the signs and symptoms and reduce the frequency of attacks.

Jane is a 35-year-old teacher. She has had sensitive skin since childhood but recently she began to develop small patches of red, scaly skin on her elbows. Initially Jane paid little attention, particularly as she noticed that they always cleared up during her holidays. When her long-term relationship ended, however, her skin condition suddenly 'exploded' and the rash now covers the whole of her arms.

Worried, Jane visited her GP who diagnosed psoriasis and prescribed medicated creams but explained that they would not prevent the rash from recurring. The doctor also referred Jane to a specialist clinic for ultraviolet treatment, but a waiting list several months long means that there is a delay here, too.

WHAT JANE SHOULD DO

Jane should make sure that her diet contains plenty of sunflower oil, olive oil or other cold-pressed oils. These contain a high percentage of polyunsaturated fatty acids which are important for a healthy skin. A friend at work advised Jane to visit a herbalist who recommended evening primrose oil capsules. The herbalist also tried to balance Jane's metabolism and improve her overall health with gentle bitters, diuretics and alterative herbs including nettle, dandelion root and leaf, heartsease and figwort. Jane should expect her condition to become worse initially, as her metabolism adjusts. A rich cream made from infused oils of marigold and cleavers applied daily will also help.

Action Plan

LIFESTYLE
Choose the seaside for your holiday destination if you can. Sunshine, swimming and long walks on the beach will help your skin to recover.

HEALTH
Visit a herbalist to discuss a holistic approach to the problem, addressing stress and emotional problems.

EMOTIONAL HEALTH
Look at underlying emotional factors. Talk to a counsellor and instigate daily relaxation techniques.

LIFESTYLE
Sunshine and sea water are beneficial for psoriasis and will help relieve the immediate symptoms. Dietary changes will also help.

HEALTH
Conventional treatments can relieve symptoms but general good physical and emotional health is the best way to help to stave off the triggers of psoriasis attacks.

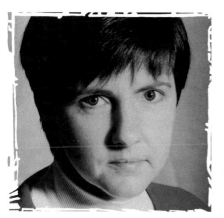

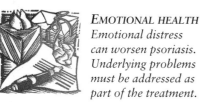

EMOTIONAL HEALTH
Emotional distress can worsen psoriasis. Underlying problems must be addressed as part of the treatment.

HOW THINGS TURNED OUT FOR JANE

After the first two weeks of herbal treatment, Jane's skin became very red and itchy. Jane found this difficult to cope with, but drinking lime flower tea, in addition to her prescribed herbal medicines, helped her with the emotional distress. Jane also discovered that she needed to apply the cream frequently at first, up to five times a day, to get relief. Two months after the initial treatment, however, Jane's condition is improving.

Hair loss treatments

The best herbal treatments are hair lotions that stimulate blood flow to the scalp and the roots of the hair. Increased circulation provides the hair with nutrients which help it to grow.

A traditional recipe for a hair lotion includes 1 ml (20 drops) of rosemary essential oil, 1 ml (20 drops) of lavender essential oil, 30 ml (1 fl oz) of nettle tincture mixed with 70 ml (2⅓ fl oz) of water. Massage well into the scalp at night. This lotion may be used long-term.

eczema are allergic reactions while others may be inherited, although both are notoriously difficult to treat. The underlying cause should be identified and treated whenever possible. Herbal medicine always combines external preparations for the skin with internal treatment. Traditional herbal remedies are alteratives like burdock, cleavers, figwort, heartsease and nettle which improve the general health of the body. If the eczema is associated with nervous tension, nervines – nerve relaxants – such as oats and lime flowers should be included. Herbal treatment for eczema is always long-term and the herbs may be taken as teas or tinctures – use standard doses (see page 84).

Herbs like chickweed, marigold and burdock can be used externally to soothe the irritation. Peppermint may be added if the skin is very itchy. The herbs can be made into creams or be used as infused oils and applied to the affected parts several times a day. For very weepy eczema, make a strong tea from walnut leaves and apply this as a compress twice a day. Let the skin dry naturally and then apply a light marigold or chickweed cream.

DANDRUFF

In this often itchy condition of the scalp, the top layer of the skin sheds its dead cells at a faster rate than normal. The old skin is seen as white flakes in the hair and on the sufferer's clothes.

Most skin problems are a sign that the body is not in the best of health. In this case, too much junk food and a lack of vitamins and polyunsaturated oils in the diet often contribute to the problem.

Internal herbal treatment should include bitter herbs like dandelion or gentian to encourage elimination of toxins. Herbalists also include alterative herbs such as nettle and burdock. A good combination is a tincture made from equal parts of dandelion leaf and root, nettle and figwort, taken in standard doses over long periods.

For immediate improvement, while waiting for internal treatments to take effect, mix together 30 drops each of sandalwood and rosemary essential oils with 50 ml (2 fl oz) almond oil. Shake well and massage into the scalp. Leave for half an hour, then shampoo out. Repeat every time you wash your hair. It is very important to rinse your hair thoroughly after using the oils to remove any loosened skin cells from it.

HAIR LOSS

Hair constantly regenerates itself and losing a small amount is normal. Abnormal hair loss, however, may be due to poor general health, stress or genetic factors.

Unfortunately, if hair loss is hereditary there are few herbal treatments that have been proven to help. For hair loss that is due to poor health or stress, herbalism can certainly offer help, see left.

HERBS FOR YOUR HAIR TYPE

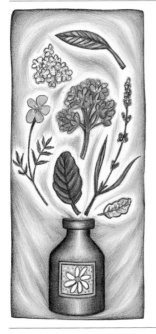

Herbs can have a dramatic effect on the health of your hair. Some preparations can help control common problems such as dandruff, while others can enhance the natural colour of your hair. Specific hair type problems, such as blonde hair being particularly fine, can also be relieved with a selection of herbal hair rinses.

HAIR TYPE	SUGGESTED HERBS
Fair	Camomile, calendula, elder flowers, mullein, rhubarb root (powdered), saffron, turmeric, yarrow
Dark	Comfrey, marjoram, nettle, parsley, raspberry leaf, rosemary, sage, southernwood, thyme
Red	Marigold flowers, red hibiscus, red oak bark (ground to a powder), ginger, saffron
Grey	Betony, marjoram, nettle, rosemary, sage, walnut
Greasy	Geranium, lavender, lemon balm, parsley, peppermint, rosemary, white dead nettle, witch hazel
Dry	Burdock root, calendula, camomile, comfrey, elder flowers, lavender, marsh mallow, sandalwood
Dull	Calendula, fennel leaf, parsley, rosemary, southernwood, stinging nettle
Dandruff	Basil, burdock root, cleavers, cypress, lavender, mint, nettle, parsley, rosemary, southernwood
Thinning	Bay, camomile, cedarwood, clary sage, cypress, horsetail (stems and branches), southernwood

EAR AND EYE PROBLEMS

It is important that any loss of hearing or impairment of vision is treated by your doctor. Some milder disorders, however, respond well to herbal remedies.

Ailments of the ears and eyes can be highly disturbing and painful. Some simple problems can have more serious side effects. Earache, for example, can cause balance problems, whilst inflammation of the eyelids can affect vision as the eyelids swell.

ACUTE EARACHE
Acute earache is a symptom of an infection of the middle ear or the ear canal. Acute ear infections need to be treated internally with immune stimulating herbs like echinacea, goldenseal or garlic. Take 1 teaspoon of tincture up to four times a day until the infection has cleared. Goldenseal stimulates the muscles of the womb and should not be taken by pregnant women.

CHRONIC EARACHE
Some people have very sensitive ears that become painful during cold and windy weather. Chronic earache may also be caused by too much catarrh in the middle ear which must be treated with anticatarrhal herbs like elderflower and eyebright. A tincture made from the herbs should be taken over several months.

Mullein oil or plain olive oil may be used to treat chronic earache. Use a few drops of the warm oil (see box) in the ear canal in cold weather to protect the ear drum.

CONJUNCTIVITIS
Inflammation of the conjunctiva, the delicate lining of the eye, causes redness, itching and weeping. This inflammation may be due to hay fever, irritation through dust or sand, or an infection. Conjunctivitis responds well to external treatment with herbal remedies.

Combine eyebright and fennel and make a strong infusion. Strain this well before use to prevent further irritation of the eye. Add a pinch of salt and use as an eye lotion, gently bathing the eyelid several times a day with a pad of cotton soaked in the mixture until the condition has improved.

INFLAMMATION OF THE EYELIDS
Allergies or infections that affect the eyelids may cause conjunctivitis-like symptoms, but there is usually pus around the eyelid which becomes very tender as a result.

Warm compresses soaked in a strong infusion of camomile are an effective treatment. Camomile has a strong anti-inflammatory action on the skin and various studies have found it to be both antiseptic and analgesic. Treat the infected eyelid frequently throughout the day with camomile compresses until it has improved.

HOME-MADE EAR DROPS

To relieve earache, use a few drops of infused oil of mullein flowers in the ear. Add 1 drop of essential oil of clove if the pain is severe. Never use external remedies on a perforated ear drum – if in doubt, consult your doctor before self-treatment.

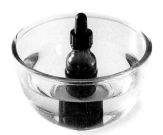

1 *Stand a bottle of oil with a dropper lid in a bowl of warm water for 10–15 minutes.*

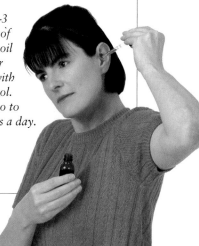

2 *Put 2–3 drops of the warm oil in each ear and seal with cotton wool. Repeat two to three times a day.*

MOUTH, TEETH AND THROAT PROBLEMS

Herbal remedies can offer widespread and effective relief from a variety of disorders affecting the mouth, teeth and throat, from catarrhal bad breath to mouth ulcers to a sore throat.

Diet plays an important part in the health of the mouth and teeth. A diet high in sugar, for example, can lead to mouth soreness, ulcers and tooth decay. Infections are the most common throat problems, although chronic ailments may be symptoms of serious underlying disorders which should be properly diagnosed before herbal treatment is applied.

BLEEDING GUMS
Sore and bleeding gums are signs of gum disease. Gingivitis, or inflammation of the gums, is one of the most common infections of the mouth. It may be caused by poor oral hygiene and a high-sugar diet.

Sage is the most popular herb for treating bleeding gums because of its astringent and antibacterial properties. Studies in Germany have confirmed its effectiveness for the treatment of bacterial and viral infections in the mouth, including gingivitis. A strong infusion of sage should be used as a mouthwash three times a day for as long as the infection persists. Other astringent herbs used in this way include marigold and witch hazel. When using witch hazel make a decoction from the dried bark.

COLD SORES
The small, weeping blisters on the lips known as cold sores are caused by the herpes simplex virus. An attack may be triggered when the body's resistance is low, for instance during a cold or at times of high or prolonged stress.

Cold sores must be treated both internally and externally. Herbs to boost the immune system, such as echinacea and St John's wort, should be taken at the first sign of a blister – 5 ml tincture, three times a day – until the infection passes.

A cream made with essential oil of lemon balm and infused oil of St John's wort will help to heal the cold sore externally. Studies carried out on lemon balm as a cold sore remedy have found antiviral properties which are confirmed in herbal practice. Apply the cream frequently throughout the day until the infection has cleared.

TOOTHACHE
A symptom of tooth decay, toothache must be treated by a dentist. Herbs can help to relieve acute toothache, but the underlying cause must be addressed. A traditional cure is to chew a clove as the essential oil is a strong analgesic and antiseptic.

A popular modern variation is to apply a small piece of cotton wool soaked in clove oil to the painful tooth and leave it there until the pain subsides (see page 45).

BAD BREATH (HALITOSIS) Although bad breath can be overpowering and embarrassing it is easily treatable. It can often be a sign of poor oral hygiene, digestive problems, bad diet, or a mouth or throat infection.

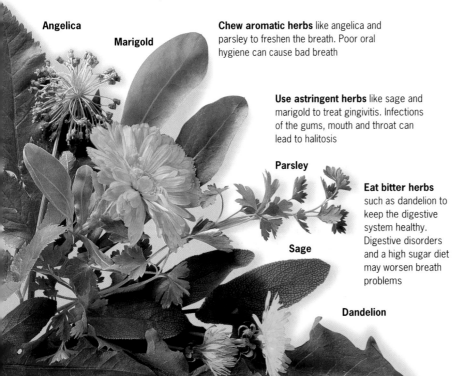

Angelica

Marigold

Chew aromatic herbs like angelica and parsley to freshen the breath. Poor oral hygiene can cause bad breath

Use astringent herbs like sage and marigold to treat gingivitis. Infections of the gums, mouth and throat can lead to halitosis

Parsley

Eat bitter herbs such as dandelion to keep the digestive system healthy. Digestive disorders and a high sugar diet may worsen breath problems

Sage

Dandelion

SAGE VINEGAR FOR A SORE THROAT

Macerating herbs in vinegar for medicinal use is an established kitchen tradition. This remedy for sore throats combines the astringent and antiseptic properties of sage with the anti-inflammatory action of vinegar. Dilute one part sage vinegar with two parts water, add a pinch of salt and gargle three times a day until the condition improves. Alternatively, soak a clean handkerchief in the solution and wring out excess liquid. Wrap the compress firmly around your throat and cover with a clean tea towel. Renew after 15 minutes. Repeat three times a day.

Ingredients
2 large sprigs of fresh sage or
   1 tbsp of the dried herb
425 ml (¾ pint) of cider vinegar

1 Loosely fill a glass jar with the fresh or dried herb. If you are using fresh sage, chop it coarsely before adding the vinegar in order to help to release the active ingredients. Don't pack the herbs in, the vinegar needs to get between the leaves.

2 Gently heat the cider vinegar over a low heat until it reaches body temperature. Pour it over the sage until the herb is completely covered and seal with a tight-fitting lid.

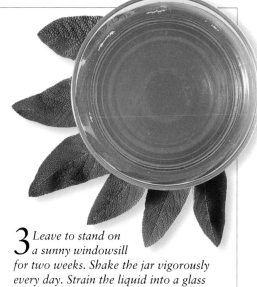

3 Leave to stand on a sunny windowsill for two weeks. Shake the jar vigorously every day. Strain the liquid into a glass bottle and stopper well. Label and date. Stored in a cool dark place it will keep for up to one year.

DENTAL PLAQUE

A build-up of dental plaque is the result of poor oral hygiene. Dental plaque encourages the growth of bacteria which cause tooth decay. Choose a toothpaste that contains astringent and anti-inflammatory herbs such as sage, peppermint, camomile and echinacea. The addition of salt or bicarbonate of soda makes a toothpaste mildly abrasive which helps to reduce plaque.

MOUTH ULCERS

Painful mouth ulcers are a sign of a low immune system and commonly occur after a cold or during emotionally stressful periods.

Marigold and myrrh are popular remedies. Herbal practice has shown them to be very effective, possibly due to their antiseptic and anti-inflammatory properties. Dilute tinctures in water (1 part tincture to 4 parts water) and use as a mouthwash three times a day until the ulcers have cleared.

Herbs that stimulate the immune system, such as echinacea, should be taken internally. Take 1 teaspoon of the tincture up to four times a day until the ulcers clear up.

SORE THROAT

A sore throat is often a minor, but extremely annoying condition caused by the streptococcus bacteria or by bacterial infections like tonsillitis or laryngitis. The throat feels very hot and swallowing can be difficult. Herbal treatment for sore throats consist of gargles and compresses and can be highly effective. If the symptoms of a sore throat last for more than three days, it is often better to consult a doctor than continue self-help. If, however, it is only a mild sore throat, accompanying a cold for example, then the following herbal preparations may help to speed recovery.

A demulcent herb like marshmallow makes a very effective remedy to soothe a sore throat. A cold infusion made from the leaves of the plant should be used as a gargle three to four times a day until the condition has improved. Add astringent and antiseptic herbs such as sage, myrrh and marigold to heal the underlying infection.

Drink sage and marigold tea to soothe any inflammation and to help your tonsils to recover from infections. You can use the tea as a gargle and drink a cup of the infusion three times a day until the infection clears.

Cider vinegar compresses are an old kitchen remedy for sore throats. Add one part of vinegar to three parts of lukewarm water and apply externally as a compress. Repeat three times a day until your sore throat improves.

Vinegar compresses will help to draw out heat and reduce inflammation in your throat. They are useful if the throat feels very hot, tender and swollen. Use a compress in addition to gargling if possible. The joint treatment should help to relieve the pain of a sore throat very quickly.

HEADACHES AND MIGRAINES

Muscular tension, eyestrain and allergic reactions can all be responsible for a headache or migraine. Herbal remedies offer relief from the pain and nausea that may accompany headaches.

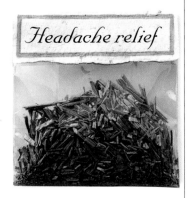

Vervain compress
For quick and gentle relief from mild headaches make a cold compress from an infusion of vervain and apply to the forehead and the back of the neck until the headache clears.

In many instances a headache can be avoided. If you know that cheese or oranges bring on pain, simply do not eat them. If your headaches are brought on by muscular tension, you should work to correct your posture and practise relaxation techniques. If your headache is already upon you, however, herbalism can offer a range of pain-relieving remedies.

HEADACHE

Headaches that are caused by nervous tension rarely follow a recognisable symptom pattern, although there is usually muscle tension in the shoulders and neck. Relaxing and calming herbs can be used internally and externally to treat nervous headaches.

Gentle relaxants such as camomile and lemon balm make very useful long-term remedies because of their sedative and antispasmodic properties. They are best taken as teas and should be drunk throughout the day. One cup at night will also aid sleep.

Essential oil of lavender has a mild sedative action which is especially effective if used in a warm bath or in an essential oil

Pathway to health

Headaches that are brought on by stress or tension can be relieved with many natural remedies. You can enhance the beneficial effect of herbal remedies by practising relaxation and visualisation techniques, such as picturing yourself floating in warm water. The release of tension together with the herbal remedies will quickly ease your headache.

burner. A warm bath enhances the relaxing effect of this plant on muscles and nervous system. Use lavender oil sparingly, adding only 5–6 drops to a bath – large doses may have the opposite effect.

Headaches that are triggered by food or drink can often be relieved with the relaxant and mildly sedative herbs mentioned above. Any lasting headache following a blow to the head should be examined by your doctor.

MIGRAINE

Migraine headaches are often accompanied by nausea, vomiting, visual disturbance and sensitivity to light; attacks can last for hours or even days.

Factors that can trigger a migraine are numerous and include foods such as cheese and chocolate, weather changes and stress. In all cases the cause of the underlying problem should be identified before any long-term treatment is decided upon.

Feverfew is an excellent herb for migraine relief because it relaxes and dilates the blood vessels in the head which contract during an attack, causing pain. It is best to take a preparation made from the fresh herb on a regular basis as a preventative measure. You can do this by eating three or four fresh leaves with a little bread. If the leaves irritate your mouth, take the herb in the form of a tincture – 5 ml every day. Feverfew has a stimulant action on the womb and must not be taken by women during pregnancy.

Caffeine-containing plants like coffee, tea, kola and guarana are widely used to check acute migraine attacks. Although excessive doses of these herbs may actually trigger migraines, small doses are valuable for treating acute attacks.

MUSCLE PAIN

Aching muscles are a familiar symptom of strenuous exercise, bad posture or influenza. Herbal remedies can help to relieve pain and ease muscular tension.

Muscles can become painful due to overexertion which causes tiny tears and inflammation in the muscle tissue. These tears usually take two or three days to heal, but herbal oils and creams applied externally can soothe the pain and speed recovery.

Touch is a powerful healing tool and using herbal oils to massage away muscle tension is a very effective way of relieving the discomfort of aching muscles. External treatment in the form of massage oils, creams, hot compresses and baths are best for muscular pain. Infused oils made from rubefacient herbs like mustard or cayenne pepper also make very good massage oils or can be added to a base cream. Alternatively, mix essential oils into an infused oil to enhance and tailor their effects.

BEFORE A MASSAGE

Take a warm bath to relax and loosen tense muscles. Add invigorating herbs such as rosemary, thyme or eucalyptus essential oils to the bath water. This stimulates the circulation and prepares the muscles for external treatment. It is easier to apply a cream or massage oil if the skin and muscles are supple and relaxed.

If you do not have time for a bath or just want to relieve aches and pains in your legs, soak your feet in a hot foot bath instead. Fill a deep bowl or bucket with warm water (just above body temperature is ideal), add 5 drops of essential oils such as thyme or rosemary, and bathe your feet for 10–15 minutes. This will stimulate blood flow to the legs and feet and make the absorption of oils and creams easier. A foot bath is also a

TYPES OF PAIN AND REMEDIES

Whatever the cause of your muscle pain there are herbal strategies to help. To make your own remedy for aching muscles, choose essential oils of herbs from the following categories. If muscle pains are accompanied by tenderness and swelling, try using cooling herbs like peppermint to hasten the healing process. Use the essential oil on compresses and in creams, or add it to a base oil and massage gently into the skin. If muscles ache because of an underlying cold or bout of flu, the pain is a sign that the body is working hard to get rid of toxins and metabolic waste products and you should neither mask nor hinder it. Gentle analgesic relief with massage will ease these muscular aches until time restores you to health.

Vulneraries stimulate cell growth and thus speed up tissue repair. Choose herbs like comfrey and camomile to treat any muscle and tendon damage

Stimulants or rubefacients dilate small blood vessels to stimulate circulation and relieve pain. Use rosemary, eucalyptus and clove to relieve rheumatism aches and pains

Analgesics help to reduce the pain through external application. Use St John's wort, lavender, clove, peppermint and camomile for pain caused by chronic fatigue, recently overextended muscles or flu

Anti-inflammatories fight inflammation. For pain due to recently overextended muscles and any pain with redness and swelling, use camomile, St John's wort and lavender

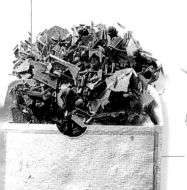
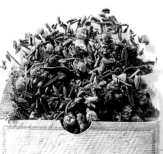
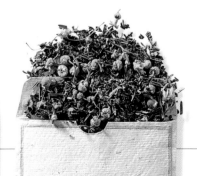
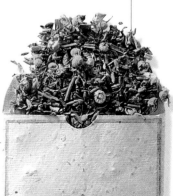

very effective way of easing the aching muscles that accompany influenza. You should not have a whole body bath while running a fever, so a foot bath is the ideal alternative.

BACK MASSAGE FOR MUSCLE TENSION

Back pain can cause mild discomfort at least, and be extremely debilitating at worst. It can also lead to other disorders such as headaches and pains in the legs and neck. Muscle tension is commonly a result of stress, bad posture or overstraining and a chronic backache can lead to many severe muscular and mobility problems.

Before you use your own massage oils for back pain, be sure that your condition is not caused by anything more serious than muscle tension, such as a prolapsed disc. If in doubt consult your doctor or osteopath, who will be able to advise you if massage is a suitable therapy for your condition.

If you are giving rather than receiving a back massage, make sure the person being massaged is warm and comfortable, then apply a hot compress over the painful area to loosen and prepare the muscles. Remove the compress before you begin to massage and use a liberal amount of oil so your hands glide easily over the skin.

With smooth, flowing strokes, work gently over the whole of the back and hips. You may increase the pressure of your strokes gradually, taking care not to cause any additional discomfort. If the person receiving the massage feels uncomfortable at any time, the massage should end.

MAKING YOUR OWN MASSAGE OIL FOR MUSCLE ACHES

An infused oil made from fresh St John's wort flowers (available from herbal suppliers) has anti-inflammatory and pain-relieving properties making it an excellent massage oil for pain relief. The addition of essential oils enhances and complements its therapeutic qualities. Both camomile and lavender have antispasmodic properties which relax muscles and help to relieve tension when used in massage. Clove oil has a strong analgesic action and is very good for muscular pain.

Ingredients
250 ml (9 fl oz) St John's wort infused oil (do not use the essential oil, which can irritate if applied directly to the skin)
5 drops lavender essential oil
1 drop camomile essential oil
2 drops clove essential oil.

1 *Pour the St John's wort oil into a clean bottle. Slowly add the essential oils, one at a time. When all the oils have been added, close the bottle tightly and shake well to blend the essential oils with the base oil.*

2 *During a massage, shake the bottle well each time you use the oil. Apply the oil liberally and work it into the skin.*

3 *It is often a good idea to have a bath or a shower before a massage to warm and loosen your muscles. Then, begin by massaging the area gently, increasing the strength of your strokes as you go along.*

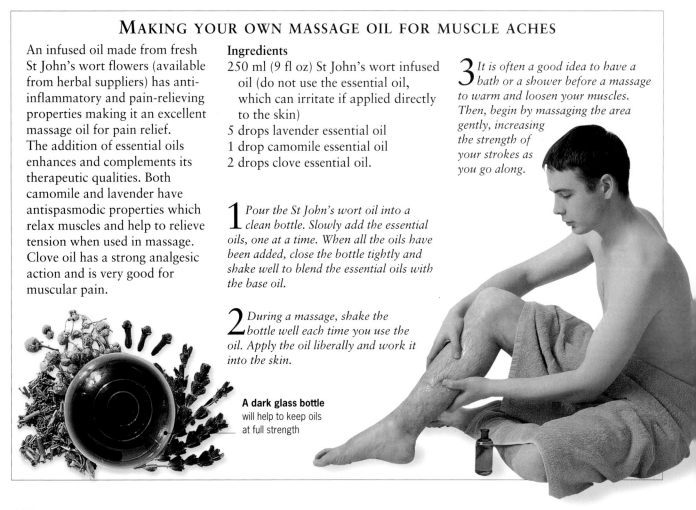

A dark glass bottle will help to keep oils at full strength

NERVOUS DISORDERS

Herbal healing can offer gentle but effective relief from the nervous, emotional and physical tensions that crop up in life from time to time.

Left unattended, problems that may be considered the simple stresses of modern living can become life-changing disorders such as insomnia and depression. It is important to deal with the minor problems of day-to-day life before they become too challenging or even defeating. Chronic pain can also lead to emotional ill-health.

ANXIETY AND INSOMNIA

Modern lifestyles produce anxiety and insomnia in many people. The symptoms include general restlessness, palpitations, lack of concentration and unspecified fears.

Many herbal remedies used to treat anxiety relax and strengthen the nervous system at the same time. Gentle nerve tonics such as camomile, lemon balm, wood betony and skullcap should be used over a long period to get the best results. They may be taken as a tea or as tinctures.

Use stronger sedative herbs for times of acute restlessness or insomnia. Valerian, passionflower and hops taken as tinctures or added to a warm (not hot) bath help to promote sleep. Hops should not be used by people who suffer from depression.

DEPRESSION

The symptoms of depression include anxiety, insomnia, loss of appetite and lack of energy. A person with depression usually has vast feelings of hopelessness.

The herb of choice to treat depression is St John's wort, a traditional remedy for nervous disorders. Recent clinical studies have also found St John's wort to be an effective antidepressant if taken internally over long periods. Scientists in Germany compare the action of St John's wort to that of MAOIs (monoamine oxidase inhibitors), a group of conventional drugs which produce stimulation in the brain and are currently used in the treatment of depression. St John's wort combines well with other nerve tonics such as lemon balm, rosemary and skullcap and can be taken as a tincture or a tea in standard doses over long periods of time (see page 84). St John's wort makes the skin more sensitive to sunlight and fair-skinned people should avoid long exposure to the sun while taking it.

STRESS

Prolonged or particularly high levels of stress cause many of today's modern illnesses, including reducing the body's immune response to infections and depleting energy levels. Unlike a virus or bacteria, the fundamental cause of stress can be difficult to diagnose, and its effects vary from person to person. This makes treatment difficult, but herbs can be used to boost both the physical and emotional responses to stress.

Recurrent infections

Physical and emotional stress can weaken the immune system and cause recurrent infections such as cold sores and upper respiratory catarrh.

Echinacea is one of the best known and most researched herbs for the immune system. It increases the body's production of white blood cells to fend off acute infections. Echinacea should be taken only for acute conditions. Taken over long periods it can overstimulate the immune system and deplete resources further. For recurrent infections take 1 teaspoon of the tincture up to four times a day as soon as symptoms appear. Only take it until the infection has cleared and then discontinue.

Mugwort may be taken in the same way as echinacea to treat acute infections but it is very bitter and must be used in small doses; 5–10 drops of the tincture up to four times a day until the condition improves. Avoid mugwort during pregnancy.

Emotional relief

Emotional problems can be triggered by many causes including stress and the problems of long-term physical pain. Holistic herbal treatment looks at the physical and emotional aspects of a problem at the same time and attempts to relieve them both.

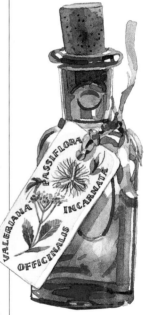

EMOTIONAL PAIN RELIEF
Tincture of willow bark taken internally has mild analgesic properties, as do many sedative herbs like passionflower and valerian. All help to support the action of external preparations used to relieve physical symptoms such as chronic pain.

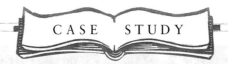

CASE STUDY

The Insomniac

The sleeplessness that insomnia sufferers experience disrupts important physical patterns and leaves the sufferer disorientated and drained of energy. This can lead to further sleep disruption if pressures from work and home build up. Herbal remedies and simple lifestyle changes can help to restore a natural and healthy sleeping pattern.

William is 39 years old and married to Pam. They have two children and recently moved house. William runs his own business and keeping it going as well as moving to a new home has been extremely stressful. He often works late and at weekends and eats on the move, although he has his main meal when he comes home at night, often around 10 pm. He is finding it increasingly difficult to go to sleep and frequently wakes in the early hours. He drinks frequent cups of black coffee throughout the day to give him energy, but now finds it almost impossible to concentrate on work. His relationship with Pam and the children has begun to suffer as he finds it harder and harder to keep an even temper.

WHAT WILLIAM SHOULD DO

William should create a timetable for his working hours leaving time for his family and relaxation. Six drops of lavender oil in a warm bath in the evening will help him relax.

William should also make sure that he has set meal times, especially in the evening. Going to bed on a full stomach may be adding to his sleeping difficulties. He should cut down on caffeinated drinks and try herbal teas of mild nerve tonics to help him relax. A good combination is camomile, lemon balm, wood betony and rosemary in equal parts. He should take 2 teaspoons of a tincture containing stronger sedative herbs, such as a mixture of valerian, passionflower and hops, half an hour before sleeping.

Action Plan

WORK
Reorganise your working day. Long working hours are not necessarily productive and often cause additional stress.

LIFESTYLE
Avoid heavy evening meals and particularly avoid eating after 8 pm. Make time to exercise each day if possible and take up some form of relaxation.

HEALTH
Herbal remedies, such as teas and tonics, can help to relax the body and calm mental and emotional states before bedtime.

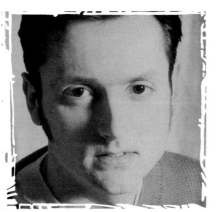

WORK
Overwork and irregular working hours can upset our natural sleeping patterns.

LIFESTYLE
Eating irregularly and having little time for exercise or relaxation can lead to sleeplessness.

HEALTH
Excessive caffeine can interrupt sleep and cause health problems in the long term.

HOW THINGS TURNED OUT FOR WILLIAM

William is now much more disciplined about his working hours – he still occasionally works weekends – and enjoys having more time to spend with his children. He replaced most of his coffee with herbal tea which he finds soothing and believes it has helped to reduce his overall stress levels. He started to sleep better after three weeks of taking the herbs and has been able to reduce the sedative tincture to 1 teaspoon every other night.

AGEING PROBLEMS

Growing old affects physical and mental abilities and reduces strength and immunity to illnesses. This can lead to general poor health and chronic disorders affecting mobility and vitality.

There are several disorders that are widely considered to be simply the normal, natural results of increasing age. Forgetfulness, loss of concentration and signs of an ageing heart, such as cold hands and feet caused by poor circulation, are common examples of ageing. The only problem with this attitude is that some people may allow their faculties to degenerate because they think it is 'their time'. For many problems of ageing, for example circulation and joint problems, there are various courses of action that can impede and prevent the growth of the problem.

CIRCULATORY PROBLEMS

It is well known that circulatory disorders are most common among the middle-aged and elderly. These emerge in two main ways as the heart muscle becomes weaker. First, the amount of blood that is pumped through the system with each heart beat lessens; second, the rate at which the heart beats increases to fulfil the body's needs. Other age-related changes involving the heart include atherosclerosis, raised blood pressure and a thickening around the valves of the heart.

To keep these disorders at bay it may help to investigate the cardiovascular properties of herbs. Some have proved highly effective in promoting adequate circulation and maintaining healthy blood pressure.

Angelica, juniper and cayenne stimulate arterial circulation and are often used to treat cold hands and feet, chilblains and some more serious circulatory disorders. Cayenne pepper is also a useful heart stimulant. Angelica and juniper should be taken as tinctures, 2–5 ml three times a day, but avoid juniper if you suffer from weak kidneys. Cayenne can be taken as a tincture, 3–4 drops, or a powder, a small pinch taken in a tea three to six times a day.

The leaves of the ginkgo tree are a valuable remedy to improve general blood circulation. Taken internally as a tincture or a tea, ginkgo can help to reduce tiredness, improve concentration and memory and give energy levels a boost. It is a slow-acting remedy and should be taken three times a day for at least six weeks before improvements begin to show.

Circulatory tonics like hawthorn and rosemary gently strengthen and regulate the function of the heart. Combined with ginkgo they can help to improve circulation to all parts of the body. Whilst hawthorn is best taken as a tincture, 2–4 ml three times a day, rosemary makes a pleasant infusion which should be drunk every day. Both herbs can be used over long periods of time with no side effects.

Ginseng has long been used as a tonic for old age. Not only does it strengthen the circulation and improve the body's overall

CHRONIC FATIGUE

Listlessness, a lack of energy and chronic fatigue may all become more common with age. There are many herbs that can help relieve fatigue but treatment should be part of general lifestyle changes to boost energy.

Ginseng is an adaptogen used to reduce stress, increase physical performance and mental abilities. It should be taken in small doses – 1 g per day, well chewed, or 10 drops of tincture twice a day – and for not more than three months to prevent side effects such as insomnia, headaches and restlessness.

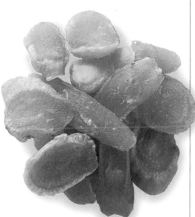

CRYSTALLINE SUPER BOOST
Ginseng is usually bought dried or crystallised, as the fresh plant is protected.

resistance to disease, it also stimulates the central nervous system. It can be either chewed raw – 1 g daily – or made into a tincture – 10 drops, once or twice every day. There is some evidence to suggest that ginseng should not be taken by people with high blood pressure and it may cause headaches if taken in large doses. Ginseng combines well, however, with other tonic herbs such as rosemary, mugwort, skullcap and wood betony.

ARTHRITIS

Rheumatoid arthritis is caused by the body's immune system reacting against the body itself, and although it can strike at any age it is particularly common among the elderly. It is characterised by swellings and deformities of the joints which can become extremely hot and painful. Osteoarthritis is caused by the wearing away of the joints and causes stiffness and pain. Internal treatment is the same for both types.

Flushing out toxins and waste products through the kidneys and liver is an important part of herbal treatment of arthritis. Alterative herbs like celery, dandelion and burdock help to keep the body free from the toxins that contribute to the condition. They are best taken as a tincture or a tea in standard doses (see page 84) over long periods of time to achieve a cumulative effect. Before aspirin became available as a drug, herbalists used the bark of the willow tree

SOOTHING ARTHRITIS
For external treatment, apply a cold compress over a hot and painful arthritic joint. The addition of a few drops of essential oil of peppermint will enhance the cooling effect. Clinical trials in Germany have found that peppermint also has a strong analgesic action if applied externally, which will provide additional pain relief. For cold, stiff joints use rubefacient massage oils such as rosemary or thyme. A herbal hand bath can be very beneficial for relieving arthritis pain.

CAUTION
While celery seeds may be used with complete safety, the isolated essential oil (apiol) of celery is toxic and should always be used with caution and never by pregnant women. Similarly, colchicum, recommended for gout, is a toxic plant that can only be prescribed by a qualified practitioner. It can cause nausea, diarrhoea and vomiting and must not be taken during pregnancy.

(see page 119) to relieve the pain of arthritis. Willow bark is most effective in this instance taken as a decoction – 3 cups daily – or taken as a tincture – 5 ml, 3 times daily. Treatment with willow bark will take a few days to begin working.

The famous English herbalist Gerard wrote in 1597 that cabbage 'is marvellous for the sinewes and joints'. Fresh cabbage, lightly crushed and applied as a poultice to a painful joint is an old kitchen remedy which is still used today. Cover the whole joint with a cabbage leaf and keep in place with a clean cotton cloth. Apply a new leaf every 20 minutes until the pain has eased.

GOUT

A disease resulting from a build-up of uric acid in the body, gout causes painful inflammation and swelling of the joints, and is most commonly found to affect the big toe.

The long-term treatment for gout is similar to that for arthritis, with a special emphasis on alterative (see page 52) herbs for the kidneys and liver, such as those mentioned for arthritis, above. A diet low in acid-producing foods is also important for successful long-term treatment. Avoid foods like sardines, anchovies, shellfish, red meat and beans. Alcohol and stimulants such as tea and coffee should also be excluded from the diet, being replaced by caffeine-free herbal teas or natural spring water.

Acute attacks of gout can be treated successfully with colchicum, a herb that is not commonly available because of its potency. Clinical research has found that it successfully prevents and relieves acute attacks of gout. Cabbage leaf poultices will help relieve the pain (see Arthritis, above).

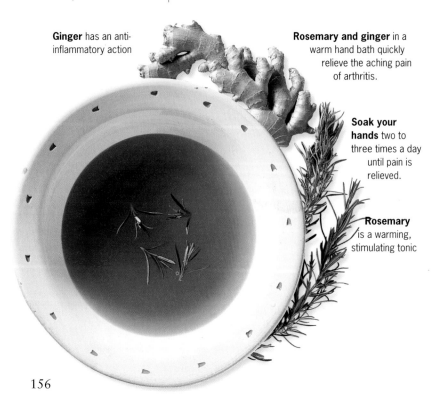

Ginger has an anti-inflammatory action

Rosemary and ginger in a warm hand bath quickly relieve the aching pain of arthritis.

Soak your hands two to three times a day until pain is relieved.

Rosemary is a warming, stimulating tonic

INDEX

A

Abortifacient 52
Achillea millefolium 85, 86
Aconite 36, 57
Aconitum napellus 57
Acorus calamus 62, 85, 87
Adaptogenic 52
Adonis vernalis 58
Aesculapius 19
Aesculus hippocastanum 42, 85, 87
Aethusa caenapium 56
Ageing problems 155–6
Agnus castus 85, 131
Agrimonia eupatoria 85, 88
Agrimony 85, 88
Alchemilla vulgaris 85, 88
Alkaloids 84
Allergic reactions 61
Allium cepa 85, 90
Allium sativum 85, 89
Aloe vera 23, 85, 90
Alpinia officinarum 85, 91
Alterative 52
Althea officinalis 85, 91
Analgesic 52
Angelica 82, 85, 92
Angelica archangelica 85, 92
Aniseed 82
Annuals 69
Anodyne 52
Anthelmintic 52
Anthraquinones 84
Anticatarrhal 53
Antiemetic 52
Anti-infective 52
Antiprotozoal 53
Antipyretic 53
Antispasmodic 53
Antitussive 53
Anxiety 153
Aperient 53
Aperitive 53
Apium graveolens 62, 85, 92
Apple 85, 113
Arctium lappa 42, 85, 93
Arctostaphylos uva-ursi 61
Aromatherapy 33
  massage 34–35
Artemisia absinthium 85, 93
  annua 46
  vulgaris 62, 85, 93
Arthritis 156
Arum maculatum 57
Aspirin 28
Asthma 138
Astringent 53
Athlete's foot 144
Atropa belladonna 57

Avena sativa 62, 85, 94
Avicenna 22
Ayurveda 38

B

Bach, Dr Edward 23, 36
  flower remedies 36
Bacteriocidal 53
Bacteriostatic 53
Bad breath 148
Barberry 25, 62
Barley 85, 107
Basil 82, 85, 115
Bath oils 42
Bay 82, 85, 111
Bearberry 61
Beech, Wooster 27
Berberis spp. 62
Berberis vulgaris 25
Betony 85, 123
Biennials 69
Bilberry 40, 85, 129
Biting stonecrop 57
Bitter orange 85, 99
Bitters 53, 84
Bittersweet 60
Black bryony 57
Black cohosh 24, 62
Black haw 85, 131
Black hellebore 57
Black horehound 134
Black pepper 82
Bladderwrack 85, 105
Bleeding gums 148
Blood root 61
Blue cohosh 24, 62
Blue flag 62
Borage 85, 94
Borago officinalis 85, 94
Box 58
Brassica oleracea 85, 96
Bronchitis 138
  thyme and eucalyptus
    inhalant 138
Broom 61
Bruising 143
Burdock 42, 85, 93
Burns 143
Buxus sempervirens 58

C

Calendula officinalis 42, 85, 95
Calluses 144
Camellia sinensis 16, 85, 96
Camomile 40, 85, 97
  tea 16
Capsella bursa-pastoris 85, 98
Capsicum minimum 62, 85, 98

Caraway 82
Cardamom 82
Carminative 53
Carrier oils 34
Cascara sagrada 61
Cassia spp. 61
Catharanthus roseus 43
Cathartic 54
Caulophyllum thalictroides 62
Caventou, Jean-Baptiste 27
Cayenne 62, 82, 85, 98
Celery 85, 92
Celery seed 62, 82
Centaurea cyanus 42
Centaury 134
Ceylon cinnamon 99
Chamomilla recutita 85, 97
Chelidonium maius 57
Cherry laurel 57
Chickweed 85, 122
Chillies 46, 85, 98
Chinese cinnamon 99
Chinese medicine 36
Chinese rhubarb 85, 117
Cholagogue 54
Choosing a practitioner 63
Chronic fatigue 155
Cicuta virosa 57
Cimicifuga racemosa 62
Cinnamon 82, 85, 99
Cinnamonum cassia 85, 99
  verum 99
  zeylanicum 99
Circulatory problems 155
Citrus aurantium 85, 99
Citrus limon 85, 100
Cleansers 40
Cleavers 85, 105
Colds 139
Cold sores 148
Coleus forskolin 46
Colic 137
Colitis 137
Colonna, Fabio 26
Coltsfoot 85, 128
Comfrey 40, 61, 85, 124
Confucius 20
Conium macalatum 58
Conjunctivitis 147
Constipation 135, 136
Convallaria majalis 59
Coriander 82
Corn dollies 46
Cornflower 42
Corns 144
Cornsilk 85, 132
Cosmetics and imagery 40
Cough 139
  thyme and coltsfoot syrup
    139
Coumarins 84

Cowbane 57
Cramp bark 85, 131
Crataegus oxyacantha 85, 100
Crateuas 20
Culinary herbs 16, 81–82
Culpeper, Nicholas 23
Curcuma longa 85, 101
Cuts 143
Cystitis 142
Cytisus spp. 61

D

Daffodil bulb 56
Daily doses 62
Dandelion 53, 82, 85, 125
Dandruff 146
Dangerous herbs 56
  identifying 56
Daphne mezereum 57
Datura stramonium 57
Daucus carota 85, 101
Deadly nightshade 57
Demulcent 54
Dental plaque 149
Depression 153
Diaphoretic 54
Diarrhoea 137
Digestive system 134–7
  leaves for 137
Digitalis purpurea 59
Digitoxin 18
Digoxin 18, 27
Dioscorea villosa 85, 102
Dioscorides 21, 26, 94
Diuretic 54
Doctrine of signatures 24, 25
Drying rack 73
Dryopteris filix-mas 57

E

Earache 147
  acute 147
  chronic 147
Ear and eye problems 147
Ear drops 147
Ebers papyrus 20, 30
Echinacea 85, 102
  angustifolia 85, 102
  purpurea 102
Eczema 144
Egrimoyne 88
Elder 85, 120
Elecampane 85, 110
Electuaries 25
Emmenagogue 54
Emollient 54
Epiphytes 44
Equisetum arvense 85, 103

Eryngium maritimum 85, 102
Essential oils 33
Evening primrose 42
Expectorant 54
Eyelid inflammation 147

—F—

Febrifuge 54
Fennel 82, 85, 104
Fenugreek 85, 127
Feverfew 26, 62, 85, 124
Figwort 62, 85, 121
Filipendula ulmaria 85, 104
Flavonoids 84
Flowering spurge 57
Foeniculum vulgare 85, 104
Foods as medicines 17
Fool's parsley 56
Foxglove 18, 59
Fuchs, Leonhart 23
Fucus vesiculosus 85, 105
Fungicidal 54
Future medicine 46

—G—

Galactogogue 54
Galangal 85, 91
Galen 21
Galium aparine 85, 105
Gall bladder problems 137
Garlic 43, 82, 85, 89
Gattefosse, René 35
Genetic engineering 44
Gentian 38, 85, 106, 134
Gentiana lutea 85, 106
Gerard, John 23, 123
Ginger 85, 132, 134
Ginkgo 46
Ginkgo biloba 30
Ginseng 61
Glycyrrhiza glabra 61, 85, 106
Goldenseal 24, 62, 85, 108
Gout 156
Grazes 143
Greater celandine 57
Green hellebore 57
Groundsel 57
Guaiacum officinale 61
Gums 84

—H—

Haemostatic 55
Hair and skin problems
    143–6
  loss 146
Hamamelis mollis 42
  virginiana 42
Hawthorn 85, 100
Hayfever 138
Headache 150
  vervain compress for 150

Helleborus niger 57
  viridis 57
Hemlock 20
Henbane 59
Herbal painkillers 45
  products 39
  skin spray 143
Herbalism and superstition 24
Herbs
  and digestive problems 52
  and emotional health 54
  and foods 82
  and general problems 55
  and minerals 17
  and Neanderthal man 19
  and nutrition 17
  and religion 38
  and respiration 55
  and Stone Age 19
  and The Biblical era 20
  and The Classical period 21
  and The East 19
  and The Middle Ages 21
  and The Renaissance 22
  and the skin 54
  and urogenic problems 53
  and vitamins 17
  and your skin type 39
  as currency 24
  as drugs 16
  as face packs 41
  as foods 16
  buying 48
  chemicals and compounds 84
  classifying by use 52
  cutting and drying 73
    barks 74
    flowers 73
    leaves 73
    roots 74
    seeds 74
  defining 16
  external preparations 51
  finding 48
  for hair types 146
  freezing 48
  growing your own 68
    from cuttings 69
    from root division 71
    from seeds 69
    in containers 72
    in pots 69
    in windowboxes 72
  internal preparations 50
  in your diet 81
  legislation of
    in other countries 50
    in UK 48
  maintaining safe levels 61
  misapplication of 61
  overdosing with 61, 62
  parts used 49
  preparing 48
  quality control 48

recommended doses of 84
retaining essential oils 51
signs of freshness 51
storing 50
therapeutic actions 52–55
treating infestation 48
when not to use 66
Hippocrates 19
Holiday herbal first-aid 135
Holistic first-aid 64
Holly 59
Homemade cosmetics 42
Homeopathy 33
Hops 62, 85, 107, 142
Hordeum vulgare 85, 107
Horse chestnut 42, 85, 87
Horsetail 85, 103
Humulus lupulus 62, 85, 107
Hydrastis canadensis 62, 85, 108
Hyoscyamus niger 59
Hypericin 109, 152
Hypericum perforatum 85, 109
Hypertensive 54
Hypoglycaemic 54
Hypotensive 55
Hyssop 85, 108
Hyssopus officinalis 85, 108

—I, J—

Ilex aquifolium 59
Ilex paraguariensis 62
Imhotep 19
Indigestion 137
Infertility 142
Influenza 139
Insomnia 153
Inula helenium 85, 110
Iris versicolor 62
Jimson weed 57
Jodrell laboratory 28
Judaeus, Isaac 26
Juniper 62, 85, 110
Juniperus communis 85, 110

—L—

Laburnum 60
Laburnum anagyroides 60
Lactuca spp. 62
Lady's mantle 85, 88
Laurus nobilis 85, 111
Lavender 42, 85, 111
Lavendula officinalis 85, 111
Laxative 55
Legendary healers 19
Lemon 40, 85, 100
  and vitamin C 17
Lemon balm 40, 42, 46, 85, 114
Leonurus cardiaca 85, 112
Levisticum officinale 85, 112
Lignum vitae 61
Lily of the valley 59
Limeflower 85, 126

Linnaeus 85
Liquorice 61, 85, 134
Liver problems 137
Lobelia 60
Lobelia inflata 60
Lords and ladies 57
Loss of appetite 134
Lovage 85, 112

—M—

Madagascar periwinkle 43
Magnus, Albertus 22
Mahonia aquifolium 85, 113
Malaria 30
Male fern 57
Malus spp. 85, 113
Mandrake 74
Mare's tail 103
Marigold 42, 85, 95
Marjoram 82
Marshmallow 85, 91, 134
Maté 62
Materia Medica 94
Mathias de l'Obel 23
Mattioli, Pierandrea 22
Meadowsweet 85, 104, 134
Melissa officinalis 42, 46,
    85, 114
Menopausal problems 140
Menstrual problems 140
Mentha
  aquatica 114
  pulegium 62
  x *piperita* 85, 114
  x *spicata* 114
Mezereon 57
Migraine 150
Mimulus 34
Mistletoe 19
Modern drug companies 43
Moisturising day creams 40
Monkshood 57
Moreton Bay chestnut 43
Morphine 27
Motherwort 85, 112
Motion sickness 134
Mountebanks 25
Mouth, teeth and throat
    problems 148–9
Mouth ulcers 149
Mucilage 84
Mugwort 62, 85, 93, 134
Mullein 85, 130
Muscle pain 151–2
  back massage for 152
  massage for 151
  massage oil, making 152

—N, O—

Narcissus pseudo-narcissus 56
Nausea 134
Nervous disorders 153

Nettle 42, 85, 128
Oats 62, 85, 94
Ocimum basilicum 85, 115
Oenanthe aquita 57
Oenothera biennis 42
Onion 85, 90
Opium 27
Oregon grape 85, 113
Orexigenic 53

—P, Q—

Pacific yew 43
Painful period sufferer 141
Panacea 25
Panax spp. 61
Papaver rhoeas 42
Paracelsus 22
Parkinson, John 23
Parsley 82, 85, 116
Parthenogenesis 88
Pasqueflower 62
Passiflora incarnata 85, 115
Passionflower 85, 115
Pelletier, Pierre-Joseph 27
Penicillin 30
Pennyroyal 62
Peppermint 85, 114
Perennials 69
Petroselinum crispum 85, 116
Pharmacognosy 30, 43
Phenolic acids 84
Physicians of Myddfai 22
Phytolacca americana 85, 116
  decandra 61
Phytomedicinals 17
Planning a herb garden 68
Plantago spp. 85, 117
Plantain (psyllium) 85, 117
Pliny 21
Poison hemlock 58
Pokeroot 61, 85, 116
Polygonatum odoratum 57
Poppy 42
Premenstrual syndrome 140
Preparations 75
  equipment 75
  external
    compresses 77
    creams 79
    infused herb oils 80
    liniments 80
    lotions 80
    ointments 79
    poultices 79
  internal 75
    capsules 77
    decoctions 76
    infusions 75
    inhalants 77
    syrups 76
    tinctures 76
  making
    compresses and poultices
      77

creams and ointments 79
  inhalants 78
  liniments and lotions 80
  vapour rub 78
  other 80
Prostate enlargement 142
Protozoa 30, 95
Prunus laurocerasus 57
Psoriasis 144
Pulsatilla spp. 62
Purgative 55
Purple coneflower 102
Quacks 25
Queen's delight 62
Quinine 27

—R—

Ragwort 57
Rainforests 44
Raspberry 85, 119
Recurrent infections 153
Red clover 85, 127
Relaxant 55
Reproductive and urinary
  problems 140–2
Respiratory system 138–9
Rhazes (Abú Bahr Mohammad
  ibn Zakarijá ar-Rázi) 22
Rheum palmatum 85, 117
Rosa spp. 85, 118
Rose 40, 85, 118
Rosemary 42, 82, 85, 118
Rosmarinus officinalis 42,
  85, 118
Rubefacient 55
Rubus idaeus 85, 119
Rue 62
Ruta graveolens 62

—S—

Sage 40, 62, 82, 85, 121
Salix alba 85, 119
Salvia officinalis 62, 85, 121
Salycilin 28
Sambucus nigra 85, 120
Sanguinaria canadensis 61
Saponin 84
Sassafras 62
Sassafras albidum 62
Scrophularia nodosa L. 62,
  85, 121
Scutellaria galericulata 85, 122
  lateriflora 122
Sea holly 85, 103
Sedative 55
Sedum acre 57
Self-diagnosis 63, 64, 66
  and chest pains 64
  and children 66
  and emergencies 66
  and headaches 66
  and protracted symptoms 66

and serious symptoms 66
  and skin problems 64
  and vomiting 64
Senecio jacobaca 57
Senecio vulgaris 57
Senna 61
Sertürner 27
Sexual impotence 140
Shaman 23
Shampoos and conditioners 42
Shepherd's purse 85, 98
Skin preparations 39, 40
Skullcap 85, 122
Socrates 20
Solanum dulcamara 60
Solomon's seal 57
Solvents 18
Sore feet 144
Sore throat 149
  sage vinegar for 149
Spearmint 85, 114
Sphagnum moss 30
Squaw vine 24
St Hildegarde 22
St John's wort 85, 109
Stachys officinalis 85, 123
Stellaria media 122
Stillingia sylvatica 62
Stomach acid 135
Stomachic 55
Stress 153
Strychnine 18, 27
Strychnos toxifera 18
Styptic 55
Susruta-Samhita 20
Sweet flag 62, 85, 87
Sydenham, Thomas 23
Symphytum officinale 40, 61,
  85, 124

—T—

Tamus communis 57
Tanacetum parthenium 26, 62,
  85, 124
  vulgare 57, 61
Tannins 84
Tansy 57, 61
Taraxacum officinale 85, 125
Taxus baccata 60
  brevifolia 43
Tea 16, 81, 85, 96
  for a fever 55
  mint and lemongrass 63
Thomson, Samuel 27
Thornapple 57
Thrush 142
Thuja 62
Thuja occidentalis 62
Thyme 82, 85, 126
Thymoleptic 55
Thymus serpyllum 126
  vulgaris 85, 126
Tibetan medicine 38
Tilia europea 85, 126

Toners 40
Toothache 148
Trifolium pratense 85, 127
Trigonella foenum-graecum
  85, 127
Turmeric 82, 85, 101
Tussilago farfara 85, 128
Tzu-I Pên Tshao Ching 20

—U, V—

Ulcers 135
Unani 38
Urtica dioica 85, 128
Vaccinium myrtillus 85, 129
Valerian 26, 85, 129
Valeriana officinalis 26, 85, 129
Valnet, Jean 35
Vasodilatory 55
Verbascum thapsus 85, 130
Verbena officinalis L. 85, 130
Vermicidal 55
Vervain 85, 130
Viburnum opulus 85, 131
  prunifolium 85, 131
Viricidal 55
Virginina skullcap 85, 122
Virostatic 55
Vitex agnus-castus 85, 131
Vomiting 134
Von Linné, Carl 85
Vulnerary 55

—W—

Wall-pepper 57
Warts 144
Water dropwort 57
Water hemlock 57
Water mint 114
Weak digestion 134
Weiss, Dr Fritz 120
Western herbalism 32
Wild cabbage 85, 96
Wild carrot 85, 101
Wild lettuce 62
Wild thyme 126
Wild yam 85, 102
Willow 28, 85, 119
Witchcraft 24
Witch hazel 42
Withering, William 23
Wolfsbane 57
Wormwood 62, 85, 93

—X, Y, Z—

Yarrow 85, 86
Yellow pheasant's eye 58
Yew 60
Zea mays 85, 132
Zingiber officinalis 85, 132

ACKNOWLEDGMENTS

Carroll & Brown Limited
would like to thank
Chelsea Physic Garden
Cosmetic Toiletry and Perfume
    Association, London
National Herbalists' Association of
    Australia, Morisset, NSW
Neal's Yard Remedies
Sacred Hoop Magazine
Weleda (UK) Ltd

Editorial assistants
Sharon Freed
Simon Warmer

DTP design
Elisa Merino

Photograph sources
8   Kings College School of
    Medicine/Department of
    Surgery/SPL
10 Science Photo Library
11 Paul Biddle/SPL
12 Dr Morley Read/SPL
13 Bridgeman Art Library
18 (Top) Heather Angel,
    (Bottom) David Murray/C & B
19 Oxford Scientific Films
20 (All) Bridgeman Art Library
21 (All) Bridgeman Art Library
22 (Left) Mary Evans Picture
    Library, (Right) Giraudon/
    Bridgeman Art Library
23 (All) Bridgeman Art Library
25 Mary Evans Picture Library
27 Science Photo Library
28 Tony Stone Images
30 David Murrary/C & B
35 The C W Daniel Co Ltd
43 Andrew Syred/SPL
44 Tony Stone Images
56 *Chatterton*, Henry Wallis/Tate
    Gallery Publications
58 (Top) Michael Strobing/Oxford
    Scientific Films, (Centre) John
    Glover/ Garden Picture Library,
(Bottom) G. A. Maclean/Oxford
Scientific Films
59 (Top) Geoff Kidd/Oxford
    Scientific Films, (Foxglove and
    Henbane) David Murray/C & B,
    (Bottom) Frithjof Skibbe/Oxford
    Scientific Films
60 (Top) Mike Slater/Oxford
    Scientific Films, (Lobelia) Ron
    Bass/Botanical Collection Ltd.,
    (Bittersweet) DeniBrown/Oxford
    Scientific Films, (Bottom) Tim
    Shepherd/Oxford Scientific films
68 Henk Dijkman/Garden Picture
    Library
70 Tim Griffith/Garden Picture
    Library
71 Wellcome Institute Library
87 (Bottom) Bridgeman Art Library
89 Elizabeth Rice/Bridgeman Art
    Library
90 (Top) Elizabeth Rice/Bridgeman
    Art Library
92 (Bottom) Elizabeth Rice/
    Bridgeman Art Library
94 (Top) Elizabeth Rice /Bridgeman
    Art Library
94 (Bottom) Bridgeman Art Library
97 Bridgeman Art Library
104 (Bottom) Elizabeth Rice/
    Bridgeman Art Library
107 (Top) Elizabeth Rice/Bridgeman
    Art Library
108 (Bottom) Elizabeth Rice/
    Bridgeman Art Library
111 (Bottom) Elizabeth Rice/
    Bridgeman Art Library
112 (Bottom) Elizabeth Rice/
    Bridgeman Art Library
113 (Bottom) Elizabeth Rice/
    Bridgeman Art Library
114 (Bottom) Elizabeth Rice/
    Bridgeman Art Library
115 (Top) Elizabeth Rice/Bridgeman
    Art Library
118 (Bottom) Elizabeth Rice/
    Bridgeman Art Library
118 (Top) Bridgeman Art Library,
119 (Top) Elizabeth Rice/Bridgeman
Art Library
120 Elizabeth Rice/Bridgeman
    Art Library
121 (Top) Elizabeth Rice/Bridgeman
    Art Library
124 (Bottom) Bridgeman Art Library
126 (Top) Elizabeth Rice/Bridgeman
    Art Library
127 (Top) Bridgeman Art Library
129 (Top) Elizabeth Rice/Bridgeman
    Art Library
130 (Bottom) Elizabeth Rice/
    Bridgeman Art Library
132 (Top) Elizabeth Rice/Bridgeman
    Art Library

Botanical illustrators
Pam Baldaro
Angelika Elsebach
Sarah Fuller
Will Giles
Sandra Pond
Ann Winterbotham

Illustrators
John Geary
Nicola Gregory
Sarah Venus
Anthea Whitworth

Photographic assistants
M-A Hugo
Mark Langridge

Hair and make-up
Kim Menzies

Picture research
Sandra Schneider

Research
Steven Chong

Index
Laura Price

75-008-01

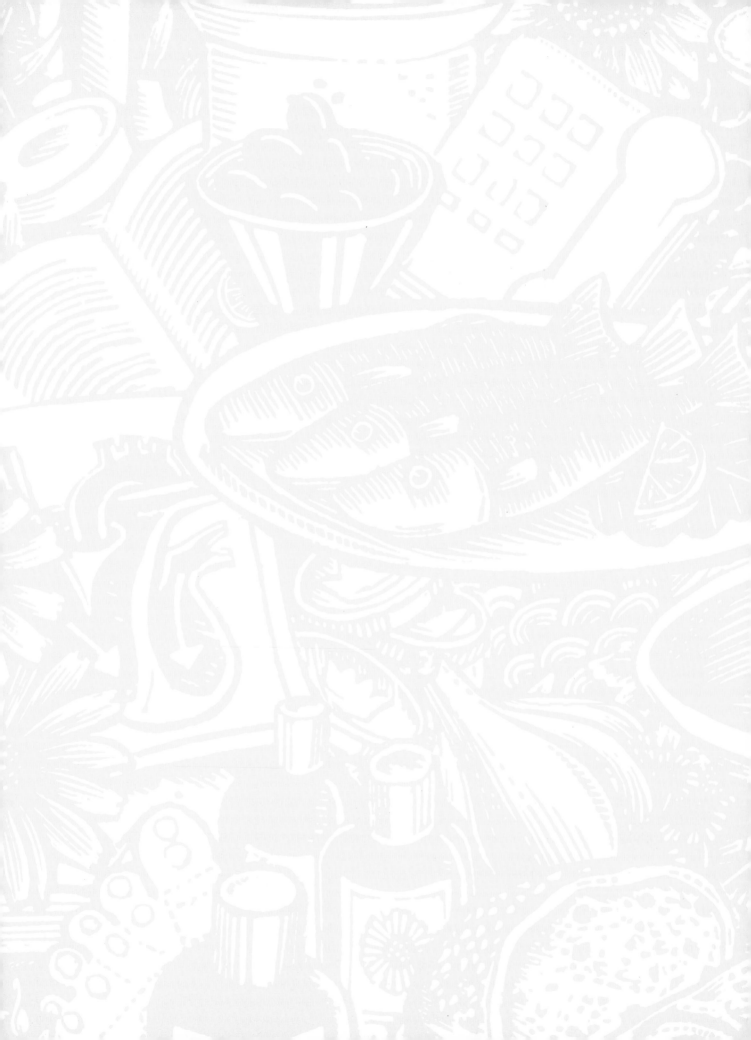